Diet Simple

Shed Pounds
Without Even Trying!

DIET SIMPLE

154 Mental Tricks,
Substitutions,
Habits &
Inspirations

Katherine Tallmadge, MA, RD

LifeLine
Press

A Regnery Publishing Company • Washington, D.C.

Cataloging-in-Publication Data on file with the Library of Congress

ISBN: 0-89526-185-5

Published in the United States by
LifeLine Press
A Regnery Publishing Company
One Massachusetts Avenue, NW
Washington, DC 20001

Visit us at www.lifelinepress.com

Distributed to the trade by
National Book Network
4720-A Boston Way
Lanham, MD 20706

Printed on acid-free paper
Manufactured in the United States of America

10 9 8 7 6 5 4 3

BOOK DESIGN BY JULIE LAPPEN
ILLUSTRATIONS BY JANE MJOLSNESS

Books are available in quantity for promotional or premium use. Write to Director of Special Sales, Regnery Publishing, Inc., One Massachusetts Avenue, NW, Washington, DC 20001, for information on discounts and terms or call (202) 216-0600.

table of contents
Diet Simple

PART 3: FAST AND DELICIOUS
BATCH RECIPES
FROM THE BEST CHEFS

APPENDIX: WEIGHT-LOSS BASICS

Introduction
Why I Wrote This Book

I first started thinking about weight problems when I was a child in Ohio. One evening, everyone but my mother was at the table eating dinner. When I rushed into the kitchen to find her, I must have startled her. She had been weighing peas on a kitchen scale, but now the peas were spilling all over the floor. I helped her pick them up.

"Mom, what are you doing?" I asked. Weighing peas, after all, seemed like a very strange thing to do.

"I'm fat," she replied. She sounded upset. "I'm fat, I'm on a diet, and I have to lose weight."

Now, you have to understand that my mother was—and is—a beautiful Swedish woman. She married an American serviceman, my father, in France, and they moved to the United States when I was 18 months old. She was definitely a star—"the Swedish beauty"—wherever we lived. Friends referred to her as another Ingrid Bergman. That certainly was the way her admiring daughter saw her.

Yet here she was, weighing peas! And that's the way it was going to be throughout her life: a constant struggle to lose 20 pounds, regain it, plus more. Every time she went on a diet and lost weight, she'd gain back even more each time. It was a constant, demoralizing, losing battle. Her problem with weight began after her third child was born (my comment "Another stinkin' brother!" became neighborhood legend). Mom had a winning personality that included a fun, goofy side. She enjoyed lots of friends, and was also artistic. Everyone, then and now, loved her. But all she could focus on was how FAT she was. The shame and disappointment that she felt was something that stayed with me.

Years later, when faced with choosing a major in college, I picked dietetics. I wasn't even aware of the inner voices affecting me at that time, of the reasons why I made that choice. It's only now, after years of reflection, that I realize why I'm so passionate about my work. I chose this as my life's vocation so that I could help people like my mother.

Like Mother, Like Daughter

Studies have shown that when parents are obsessed with weight problems, their children are also more likely to have weight problems in life. And when parents are not consistent in their attitudes toward food—when they alternate constantly between "off" and "on"—the children are more likely to develop eating disorders.

In my case, overeating became a way of life when I left home for college. I stuffed myself with sweets, chips, and other snack foods—all of the things I couldn't get that easily at home, but which now were readily available.

Visiting my Swedish grandparents one summer didn't help. We would start the day with a big breakfast bowl of strawberries—nothing wrong with that so far, but wait—with heavy cream *poured* over them. We'd end the evening with cookies and hot chocolate—made with cream, naturally. And I wasn't exactly starving between breakfast and bedtime. I cringe when I see a photo of me, standing between my grandparents, that was taken between my sophomore and junior years. With those chipmunk cheeks, I was a regular Swedish meatball!

My weight problem in college followed the classic yo-yo pattern. I'd gain weight, diet, gain the weight back, diet again, and so on. Eventually I had a full-blown eating disorder. I was shocked at my own behavior, and sought help immediately.

I realize now that my eating disorder was a grief reaction to the death of my American grandmother, which left a great void in my life. It was also a result of a childhood spent with a mother with a poor body image who was constantly dieting. It was a very difficult time in my life, both personally and professionally.

I knew that my scientific knowledge of nutrition wouldn't be enough to solve my problems. I decided to pursue a master's degree in behavioral science because I had come to realize that our *behavioral* patterns lead to our physical problems. I wanted to learn how to change people's lives, including my own.

The bottom line, dear reader, is that I'm no sacrosanct preacher looking down at a congregation of sinners. I've *been* there! I've been overweight. I had a weight problem and an eating disorder. And I know what it takes to come back from those depths of despair—and to stay on top!

It Will Work for You

My professional career has evolved in response to my desire to make a real difference in people's lives. I quickly realized, as a college intern with the National Institutes of Health, that a hospital setting was not for me. You meet most patients only once, and hand them a nutritional print-out. Minimal impact, there. I longed to spend more time with them, but there weren't enough hours in the day to counsel the patients in the hospital.

Only marginally more satisfying was the year I spent managing the dietary program of a large nursing home. I needed this experience in order to get my certification as a registered dietitian—it was, in effect, a professional internship. But while I hired, trained, and managed a crew of 20, and was in charge of 130 patients' nutritional health, I wanted more personal interaction with those patients. And, I knew that their nutritional problems had begun long before they arrived at that nursing home.

I soon realized that private practice was the only path that would give me the opportunity to help people turn their lives around. That was a scary move—my first year, I earned all of $4,000!—but I survived, and referrals from the doctors I worked with helped me build my practice to a sustainable level.

Watching my clients change negative patterns of behavior into positive ones has been a joy, and I've felt honored to be a part of that process. In particular, I enjoy hearing clients tell me that they never knew that losing weight could be so easy, or so positive. Many clients actually sit in my office saying, "It can't be this easy. Tell me that there's something more difficult I have to do." That's music to my ears!

I've also learned from my clients. In fact, most of the strategies in this book come from them, at least indirectly. When I give them suggestions, they invariably make changes and adaptations that work best for them. When I saw how a series of small, positive steps could lead to significant accomplishments, it seemed only natural to let others in on those secrets—first with articles in popular and professional publications, then with television and radio appearances, and now with this book.

I've done it. My clients have done it. And now you can too!

Part 1

The Diet Simple *Promise*

1

Easier Than You Think

Every year, publishers churn out dozens, if not hundreds, of diet and weight-loss books. Pick up any newspaper or magazine, and you're likely to see a few articles devoted to healthy eating and dieting.

I don't think it's an exaggeration to say that Americans have an insatiable appetite (forgive the pun) for information about losing weight. This is a good thing, in a way. Overweight and obesity are among the leading risk factors for dozens of chronic, serious health threats.

Then there are the social costs. In a society that celebrates thin, those of us who struggle to control our weight often feel marginalized, at best. If the plethora of weight-loss information helps even a few people lose weight, the cost of paper and ink seems well justified.

Alas, most of the people who read these books and articles won't lose much weight—and they'll be even less likely to keep it off permanently. Americans, regrettably, are getting heavier by the year. In fact, more than half of American adults (61 percent, to be exact) are overweight, and nearly a quarter are obese.

I've known a few people who woke up one day, stood in front of the mirror, and said to themselves, "This is it, I'm going to lose weight"—and actually succeeded the first time. But they're the exceptions. The overwhelming majority of those who try to lose weight will have a lot of false starts. They might lose weight for awhile, but the weight slowly comes back. They're always switching diet plans—sometimes a new one each month. They take weight loss supplements. They eat more fiber, more protein, more whatever—and the darned weight still won't budge.

It doesn't have to be this way. Losing weight isn't rocket science (even though a lot of big-name authors, with their infinitely complex plans, would like you to believe it is). It doesn't require memorizing long lists of foods and calorie contents. You don't have to quit eating chocolate or pumpkin pie. You don't even have to "diet" in any formal way. In fact, the less you diet, the more successful you're going to be.

The Elephant in the Living Room

About 30 seconds after starting my practice as a weight loss and nutrition counselor, I began hearing stories from clients about promising diet programs that went bad. It was puzzling. Some of the approaches, at least the ones I was familiar with, sounded reasonable. Why weren't they working?

Before I could help my clients lose weight, I had to understand where they were coming from. So I set aside some time to read the best-selling diet books. I spent weeks in the aisles of a huge bookstore in the Georgetown neighborhood of Washington, where I browsed through hundreds of books in the Diet and Nutrition section.

I began to understand the problem. Do you remember the story about the elephant in the living room? Imagine an elephant surrounded by inquisitive (and blindfolded) people. One by one, they approached the elephant, touched one particular part, and tried to identify what they were feeling. They were clueless!

That's the image that comes to mind when I think about all of the diet plans out there. Most of them focus on particular parts of the problem—calories, fat, lack of exercise, and so on. Few look at the big picture, and even fewer address the real-life situations and challenges that people find themselves in every day.

Another thing I've noticed is that many diet plans tend to insist on unnecessarily rigorous goals, along with complicated styles of eating that no sane person is going to follow for very long. All I can say is that the Puritan spirit is alive and well in the diet industry. No matter how much you want to lose weight, following these joyless programs almost guarantees failure.

Which brings us to *Diet Simple*. It's comprehensive, in the sense that I have tried to provide all of the information that you need to lose weight. But it's not complicated. Quite the opposite. My feeling is that you already know the basics: that fruits and vegetables are good, too much fat is a problem, and a little extra exercise is always nice. I'm not going to waste your time talking about things that you already know. Rather, I have provided hundreds of practical (almost mindless!) ways to incorporate smart eating and exercise in your already busy life. Diet and nutrition are the core of the program, but you'll also find a lot of tips for managing stress, getting more exercise (without *really* exercising), and controlling all of those emotional ups and downs that really put on the pounds.

You can think of *Diet Simple* as an enticing buffet of easy-to-digest tips, strategies, and mental tricks. The advice is simple, but not simplistic. And it's very goal oriented. Rather than merely asserting that particular strategies—giving up those croutons on a Caesar salad, for example—can be helpful, I took the next step and calculated the actual weight loss that you're likely to achieve.

No one is going to follow each and every piece of advice in this book. That's fine. I want you to pick and choose among them. Find the strategies that fit your personality and lifestyle. Check the amount of weight you can lose with each one. You may find that you only need a few of these tips—or a few dozen—to get your weight where you'd like it to be.

The *Diet Simple* program is easy. It's based on solid science. And because it offers such a huge menu of choices, it can be customized to match your lifestyle, habits, and appetites.

Does it work? Don't take my word for it. See for yourself!

2
Tiny Changes, Lasting Results

I f you follow the strategies in *Diet Simple*, you're going to lose weight.

How's that for confidence?

Yes, I know that every best-selling diet book and the so-called "experts" make the same claim. What makes my approach different?

For one thing, every tip in *Diet Simple* is based on sound science. I've spent a lot of years studying the different ways in which diet, exercise, behavior, and even emotions affect weight control. Drinking water before meals *will* reduce your appetite. Avoiding late-night calories *can* reduce fat storage. Allowing yourself to splurge now and then *does* improve motivation. Follow these and other tips in the book, and you're going to be successful. My experience, and the experience of the country's top experts, bear this out.

Will everyone who follows these tips succeed right away or achieve model thinness? Of course not. Losing weight requires commitment and long-lasting motivation. Some people are almost awesome in their intensity. Others need more cajoling and encouragement—and perhaps a failure or two before they're ready to go all the way.

Diet Simple accommodates both groups: those who are truly committed and want to utilize every technique available, and those who are more tentative and want to sample a variety of different options.

Here's what you'll find in the following pages:

An approach that's comprehensive, but not complicated. Diet and nutrition are at the heart of my approach, but I also stress physical activity, stress management, and behavioral techniques for coping with today's supercharged world.

Tips that are very easy to implement, and goals that are easy to achieve. You won't find a complicated, rigorous program. Rather, I focus on small, painless changes that you can make every day—and that will leave you wondering where the pounds went.

Simple Changes, Lasting Results

Nearly everyone who struggles with weight will succeed at times and fail at others. Doctors call this "weight cycling," better known as "yo-yo dieting."

For a long time, researchers believed that people whose weight cycled up and down were almost condemned to failure. It was thought that yo-yo dieting made it increasingly difficult to lose weight over time. Because nearly everyone goes through this cycle at least a few times, the news seemed discouraging.

More recently, the National Task Force for the Prevention and Treatment of Obesity reviewed some 28 medical studies on weight cycling. The conclusion: "There is no convincing evidence that weight cycling in humans has adverse effects on body composition, energy expenditure, risk factors for cardiovascular disease, *or the effectiveness of future efforts at weight loss.*"

The National Weight Control Registry has studied thousands of people who have lost at least 30 pounds (and have maintained that loss for at least a year) to determine the reasons for their success. Ninety percent of this group had failed at previous weight-loss attempts. "They tried all the wrong ways to do it," the study's authors noted, "and then they figured out the right ways to do it."

In other words, a history of yo-yo dieting has no effect on your body's ability to shed pounds. That's the good news.

The bad news is that the more often people go on diets, fall off of diets, and move on to new diets, the harder it becomes *emotionally* to succeed. This is especially true when people attempt (and fail) to lose weight with very rigorous, low-calorie diets.

I *hate* fanatical diet programs. They take the joy out of eating. Heck, they take the joy out of living! And the research is pretty clear by now that too-tough diets simply don't work for most people. Even if you lose weight initially, you're going to get bored or frustrated with all of the restrictions. Every time you go off the diet, then try it or something similarly restrictive in the future, your odds for success drop even lower, and the scientific studies bear this out.

Finally, let me present some of the findings from the bible of obesity treatment practitioners, Clinical Guidelines on the Identification, Evaluation, and Treatment of Overweight and Obesity in Adults, published by the National Institutes of Health.

Your initial goal, say the guidelines, should be to lose 10 percent of your weight in 6 months. That's a relatively modest, achievable goal which can be obtained by implementing just a handful of the suggestions in *Diet Simple*. Most of the report details the health benefits of losing weight, but here are some of the suggestions of how to reach that desirable goal:

- "Large individual variation exists.... There is, therefore, no 'cookbook' or standardized set of rules to optimize weight reduction." (Again, the individualized *Diet Simple* approach.)
- "It is better to maintain a moderate weight loss over a prolonged period than to regain from a marked weight loss."
- "Though very moderately low calorie diets produce greater initial weight losses than low calorie diets, over the long term of [more than] one year, weight loss is more sustainable with moderately low calorie diets."

This is exciting news from the experts. But I didn't need to hear it from them. My own experience from working with my clients has taught me that you don't have to go on depressing or demoralizing diets to lose weight. And the more you try, the more you learn. Your chances of succeeding are still great—even if you've tried and failed in the past.

So, for good reasons, I take a radically different approach from the diet faddists. I don't encourage people to count up every calorie they consume. I don't insist on giving up ice cream or Chinese takeout. And I certainly don't push people to sign up at their local gym, as long as they're willing to get regular exercise in some other way.

What I do encourage people to do (and what I do myself) is to approach weight loss by making *many* incremental changes. Eating one less takeout meal a week. Starting the day with oatmeal. Having a snack before settling in at happy hour. These and other simple changes add up to a lot of lost calories—and weight—over the course of the year. Why go through the misery of a super-tough diet when you can make tiny changes that will have even better results?

Do Less, Gain More

The same approach that I recommend for diet and nutrition—making a series of small changes over time—also works for exercise. It's true that hard-core exercise is an excellent way to control weight. The drawback is that it's a real turnoff for most people. Jogging three miles a day will certainly burn impressive amounts of calories. But who does it? Most people find themselves thinking about jogging, not doing it, and then feeling guilty about it. Hey, that's real helpful!

What's the alternative? There are many, as it turns out. Let me summarize some recent recommendations from the Centers for Disease Control and Prevention and the American College of Sports Medicine:

- People are more likely to stick with low- to moderate-intensity physical activities than all-out workouts. In other words, taking an extra few walks around the mall might be better for losing weight than attempting—and giving up on—more rigorous types of exercise.
- Moderate physical activity is just as good for your overall health as sweating through competitive aerobics classes or other high-intensity workouts.
- You'll get excellent health and weight-loss benefits just by being active for a total of 30 minutes a day. Taking stairs instead of elevators. Walking to the corner store. Dancing. As long as it all adds up to 30 minutes—and if you do everything at about the same intensity as a brisk walk—you'll be in great shape.

Are you getting the idea? It's the same idea, really, as making small, but consistent, changes in your diet. And it's the premise of *Diet Simple*. I've found that people who make a series of small changes—so small, in many cases, that they hardly notice them—lose more weight over time than those who embark on all-or-nothing diet plans. It's also a lot more fun because they continue to live life to the fullest!

Weight loss experts agree that the initial goal should be to lose 10 percent of your weight in 6 months. That's not very much at all. It's a good goal because nearly everyone can achieve it, and when you've been successful once, you'll be more motivated to keep it up.

Unfortunately, the weight-loss industry is dominated by those who insist that the only road to weight loss is to follow absurdly detailed eating plans, or to exercise at a level that would tax trained athletes, let alone the "normal" men and women I see every day.

Terrible advice! In my experience—and the experience of today's top experts—the tortoise beats the hare every time. Look at it this way:

All or Nothing = Nothing

Slow but Steady = Victory

That's the foundation of *Diet Simple*. Set reasonable goals. Make small changes. Look for approaches that complement, not dominate, your life. You will lose weight. I guarantee it!

3
Goals You Can Live With

So many of my friends and clients have tried, with varying degrees of success, to lose weight. Why does it have to be such a difficult and frustrating process?

Part of the problem, I think, is that so many diet plans make completely unrealistic promises. Instant weight loss! Look great in 30 days! Unless you're an expert in the field, it's almost impossible to know for sure what's real and what's not—what works and what's nothing more than marketing hype.

My approach is very different. When I first meet with clients, I always emphasize that losing weight and keeping it off is a *journey*, not a once-and-done technique. I do spend a lot of time talking about calories, styles of eating, and so forth, but I'm really more concerned with attitude. Once you understand the basic issues, such as the need to eat less fat and get more exercise, successful weight loss mainly depends on motivation.

Ah, motivation—that's the hard part! It's easy to make the decision to lose weight, and it's easy to succeed for awhile. But over time, everyone's motivation tends to flag a bit, and that's when the risk of gaining—or regaining—weight becomes a real issue.

Setting Goals, Keeping Goals

I've found that the best way for people to stay motivated on their weight-loss journeys is to have very specific goals at every step of the way. Goals change all the time, of course. If you've just started thinking about your weight, your goal might be as simple as to lose a few pounds this month. Over time, your goals may shift to things like, "I want to be as physically active as I used to be," or, "I want to wear the same jeans I wore five years ago."

Goals are good. Specific goals are even better because they give you something concrete to aim for. Goals are also an excellent way to measure your progress along the way.

I can't stress enough that goals should be fun and liberating—not just another ball and chain that weighs you down and reminds you of your failures. (We all have them, believe me!)

Everyone's goals are different, of course. I don't presume to have a one-size-fits-all set of goals that works for everyone. Over the years, however, I have developed some goal-setting strategies that I think can make a real difference.

For example:

- Every goal should be your goal, not your nutritionist's, your friends', or your mother's. Unless you truly and completely want to achieve a certain goal, take it off your list.
- It should be stated positively. Don't tell yourself what you won't do. Emphasize what you will do.

- It should have a time frame. Tell yourself when you're going to start achieving a goal, and when you hope to achieve it.
- It should be realistic. Telling yourself "I will eat 100 fewer calories most nights of the week" is a realistic goal because it's one that you can reasonably achieve. Telling yourself "I'll look like I did when I was 20" is probably unrealistic.
- It should be measurable. "I want to lose 5 pounds this month" is a good, measurable goal.
- It should really matter to you. Is one of your goals to look like the aerobics lady on TV? To be able to run a marathon? To wear the new fashions? Nothing wrong with any of these, as long as they're goals you've chosen for yourself and are willing to work hard to achieve.

Your Personal Goal Worksheet

You can think of goals as interim steps on the journey to weight loss. Some goals are long term, some aren't—but all goals will serve to guide you to a particular place you want to be.

I ask all of my clients to think about where they'd like to be in one year. This sort of big-picture goal is a great way to help you choose the dozens of little goals that will help get you to where you want to be.

Do you have a pencil or a pen? Good! Let's decide where you want to be in a year.

Weight

One year from now I want to weigh _____ pounds. This will be a loss of _____ pounds from my present weight of _____ pounds.

This translates to _____ pounds per week.

Shape

What is it about my appearance that I'd most like to change by losing weight? (Examples: the size clothes I'd like to wear; losing the belly bulge; a slimmer waist or thighs; more muscles; etc.)

_____

_____

_____

Medical

One year from now I want my cholesterol to be _____.

I want my blood pressure to be _____.

I want better mobility in my (list the joints or body parts that you'd like to improve) _____.

Other health benefits I want to achieve include:

_____

_____

_____

Energy Levels

One year from now I want more and better energy. My goals include (list specifics, such as "walk with a lighter step" or "be able to spend more time with friends):

_____

_____

_____

Happiness

One year from now I want to feel better about myself in the following ways (examples: "having more confidence" or "developing more rewarding relationships"):

_____

_____

_____

Is every line filled in? Congratulations! You've made the first step toward achieving your goals: less weight, more strength, better energy—whatever you want!

Don't forget this page once you've filled it out. As the year progresses, look at it frequently. Assess your progress for each of the different goals. Add new goals or revise old ones as necessary. Think of this "goal sheet" as your roadmap for the coming year. You can change direction at any point. You can slow down or speed up. But at least you know where you're going!

Let your journey begin!

Part 2

Weight-Loss Plans That Work For You

4

Really Simple Strategies for Everyone

Especially appropriate for: _Disorganized eaters, Emotional eaters, Entertainers and socializers, Frequent travelers, Everyone else!_

O ne thing that I've learned in my many years of practice is that there isn't a single diet plan or weight-loss strategy that works for everyone. I almost go crazy when best-selling diet books or weight-loss gurus (who really ought to know better) promise success for anyone who follows _this_ plan or eats only _these_ foods. If only life were so simple!

Anyone who has struggled with weight gain knows that there is a multitude of overlapping factors that play a role. Some of them—cravings for sweets, for example—are constant, or pretty close to it. Others change as our lives change. A 19-year-old who's off to college for the first time will gain weight for entirely different reasons than a senior executive at a bank. Alcohol consumption, going out to restaurants, exercise (or the lack of it), time pressures—these are just a few of the *individual* reasons that people gain weight. I suspect there are hundreds, if not thousands, more.

It's true that many of those with weight problems can be grouped into a few very broad categories—those who don't shop regularly or plan efficiently, for example, or those who socialize or travel a great deal. When I first meet with clients, I try to get a sense of their overall life patterns because this makes it easier to devise effective strategies that will fit many, if not all, of their needs.

But I fully recognize that the reasons we gain weight are endlessly varied. You may recognize parts of yourself in later sections of this book, but I wouldn't presume for an instant that you *only* need more organization in your life, or you *only* need to control emotional eating. By all means, pay attention to those tips. They'll help you lose weight, I promise! But I'd hate to see anyone focus too much attention on a few weight-loss strategies when there are so many to choose among.

No matter what you think is the "main" reason that you've gained weight, don't skip this section! Some of the following tips can be used every day; others will apply only to certain occasions—when you're talking on the phone, for example, or settling into a booth at the neighborhood greasy spoon.

I haven't put these strategies in any particular order, for the simple reason that they're all effective. In addition, the tips in this chapter and throughout the book vary a great deal in what they ask of you. Most of the suggestions are incredibly easy to incorporate into your life. Going vinaigrette instead of "creamy" on your salads, using oil instead of butter in cooking, going "surf" instead of "turf" in restaurants—they're all very easy changes to make. And yet they still amount to lots of pounds lost.

Other tips require a bit more dedication. Getting a dog and walking it religiously is more of a life change—but one most of my clients relish. Taking up yoga or changing your environment takes a bit more time and thought, as does keeping a food diary or even editing your shopping habits. But even these changes won't be hard if you follow my advice. Whether they're right for you—at this particular time or on any particular day—you'll have to decide for yourself. Try a few of these approaches. If they're not right for you, give them up and try some different ones.

Everyone gains weight for different reasons—and everyone needs different approaches to lose it and keep it off.

Good luck—and good eating!

> **NOW it's official: You can eat a chocolate sundae every afternoon and still lose weight.**

■ ONE of my clients, Jennie, almost always snacks in the afternoon. She views these snacks as "rewards" for getting through another day of drudgery. Of course, these same snacks contribute to her weight problem.

My advice to her (and I'm pretty proud of it): Have a chocolate sundae every day.

I know this sounds strange, but here's why it helps. The chocolate syrup that you pour over ice cream isn't exactly lean, but that's okay because underneath the chocolate—the sundae part—is fresh fruit instead of ice cream. Fruit is a lot better for you than ice cream, and the chocolate provides a slightly sinful incentive to make the switch seem worthwhile.

Almost any fruit works with chocolate syrup—strawberries, bananas, peaches, take your pick. Apart from the fact that a fruit sundae is deliciously fresh tasting and low in fat, it makes a great substitute for other snacks that *really* load on the calories.

BOTTOM LINE: Lose 9–35 pounds

A tablespoon of regular chocolate syrup has about 50 calories. Pour it over fruit, and your total is about 110 to 160 calories. Compare that to the usual snacks—a candy bar, for example, has about 250 calories, and an ice cream cone has about 500—and you can see why substituting the fruit sundae can lead to impressive amounts of weight loss. Make the switch every day, and you can count on losing 9–35 pounds in a year.

PEOPLE who only exercise when they're in the mood generally don't exercise very much. The solution: Put exercise on your calendar—or set an alarm that tells you when it's time to slip on your sweats.

■ DISORGANIZED eaters tend to be intense. They work too hard, whether their work is running an office or managing a family. They focus on work so much that they find it hard to stop for meals, let alone for regular exercise.

The only way to exercise regularly is to make it an integral part of your day. But first, you have to remember it. I advise people to give themselves reminders that they can't ignore.

Maybe you're the sort who religiously keeps a calendar or a "to do" list. If so, write in an exercise session. Allow for at least 15 minutes, preferably at the same time every day. Give it the same priority that you would any other "must do" event in the day.

Don't keep a calendar? In that case, set an alarm clock, or an alarm radio tuned to an upbeat music station. Have it turn on when it's time for your daily exercise. Set the volume *loud* so you can't miss it.

BOTTOM LINE: Lose 6–14 pounds

Even a modest amount of exercise—say, walking 5 times a week for 15 minutes each time—burns a lot more calories than slaving away at the office. If you do nothing else but walk most days of the week, you can count on losing at least 10 pounds a year.

> I'M not kidding. There's no easier way to get rid of fatty leftovers than to activate your canine disposal unit. Besides, dogs need walks, and so do you!

■ LET ME tell you about Peter, a client of mine who lives in a beautiful condominium. Peter is single and has a reasonable amount of free time, but he could never work up the motivation to work out.

Recognizing that he had to get some exercise, and being fully aware of his own lethargic habits, Peter decided to get a four-legged personal trainer. He figured that having a dog would force him out of the house at least a few times a day.

So he visited the animal shelter, where he fell in love with Bitze, a cocker spaniel. Sure enough, Bitze insisted on going for walks several times a day. The two of them took long strolls along the Potomac River. The exercise felt good, and simply playing with Bitze helped Peter unwind at the end of the day.

Here's a bonus. Scientists have been looking at the links between pets and (human) health. People who spend time with their dogs, for example, can have dramatic reductions in blood pressure.

BOTTOM LINE: Lose 46–89 pounds

Peter burned about 5 calories per minute walking slowly or 9.5 calories per minute during his more brisk walks with Bitze. All totaled, he spent 90 minutes walking each day. As a result, he burned about 450–855 calories every day! Amazing what man's best friend can do.

WHEN your body feels alert, you tend to eat less. When you're physically tired or lethargic, on the other hand, it's easy to turn to food for an artificial boost.

■ NO ONE I know really enjoys stretching—but once you've done it, the surge in energy can be remarkable. One stretch I really like is the "bed stretch." You don't need workout clothes or tennis shoes to do it. As the name suggests, you don't even have to get out of bed to do it—although you may be more comfortable lying on a carpet or rug.

Lie on your back with your arms straight over your head and your legs straight. Fully stretch your arms and legs in opposite directions for 5 seconds, relax, then do it again. Imagine that you're making a "snow angel"—that's all there is to it!

This stretch uses most of your large muscle groups, including muscles in the shoulders, arms, hands, feet, and ankles. If you do it every day, your body will feel stronger and more energized. The better you feel physically, the less likely you'll be to depend on food for an energy boost.

BOTTOM LINE: Lose 7 pounds

How much will stretching affect your weight? Well, if feeling better overall helps you turn down a before-bed snack, you can count on saving about 150 calories right there. If you stretch—and avoid snacks—3 nights a week, you can count on losing at least 7 pounds. Stretch more, lose more!

> **YOU already know you should be drinking lots of water rather than soft drinks. Here are the real reasons it's so effective.**

■ ALL of those people walking around with their very own sip bottles—is anyone really that thirsty? Let's forget the trendiness for a moment: Water really is the perfect beverage when you're trying to lose weight.

I advise almost everyone to drink at least 8 full glasses of water daily. It takes up room in the stomach and acts as a natural appetite suppressant. It helps the muscles maintain good tone, and it also inhibits skin sagging that often follows weight loss. Most importantly, your body needs water to metabolize fat!

To get in the habit of drinking water regularly, go ahead and join the crowd. Stock up on one-quart plastic containers and keep them with you all the time—at work, in the car, next to your bed, and so on.

Place bottles of water in front of the refrigerator, a none-too-subtle reminder of what to reach for first.

If your tap water isn't exactly tasty, consider buying bottled spring water. Add sliced lemon, lime, or cucumber to your water. The delicious pure taste will give you yet another incentive to drink more.

BOTTOM LINE: Lose 17–22 pounds

If you are drinking a sweetened, calorie-rich soft drink every day, substituting water will add up to a lot of lost calories. Plus, the water will tame your appetite, leading to even better calorie control.

THE next time you're in a supermarket, read the label on the back of your favorite potato chips. Shocking!

■ THE AVERAGE 7-ounce serving of traditional potato chips has 1,050 calories. That's potentially more than you'd get in a healthful, three-course dinner!

I'm not suggesting giving up chips (heaven forbid). But I do recommend switching to baked chips. A 7-ounce serving has about 840 calories. It's still not lean, but it's a lot better than the fried kind. Plus, you're giving up a lot of the dangerous fat that's used in frying.

You may find that baked chips are just as tasty as the fried ones—or you may want to add a little bit of salt to bump up the taste. (If you have high blood pressure and have been told to avoid sodium, forget the extra salt.) Or serve them with nonfat salsa: You don't even notice the difference in the chips.

BOTTOM LINE: Lose 3 pounds

Let's assume you eat one bag of chips a week. Switching to baked chips could save you 10,920 calories over the course of a year. Do you enjoy chips every day? The switch will save you 76,650 calories.

Now for the clincher: For every bag of baked chips that you substitute for the fried kind, you'll be giving up 5 tablespoons of pure lard. That means that approximately 70 grams of fat won't be calling your arteries "home."

Hey! Pass the chips!

THE ways you talk to yourself influence how hopeful you are about your goals and your life. Want to lose weight? Think good thoughts!

■ IN THE PAST, whenever something exciting was on my horizon, I would immediately start worrying about things that could go wrong. Take this book. It's one of the most exciting things that has ever happened to me, but my self-talk went something like this: "If my book is successful, I may get unwanted attention and be criticized."

What does this have to do with weight loss? Everything! If your self-talk is negative, you'll almost certainly find yourself turning to food for comfort. You'll be less likely to stick with a weight-loss program, and you'll get discouraged easily. My self-destructive self-talk caused me to procrastinate for ten years before I finally finished this book.

With a combination of professional guidance and self-exploration, I gradually became aware of my thought patterns and the ways in which they were affecting—and harming—my life. Ask yourself if you often have trouble achieving the things you want most out of life. Is it possible that you're subconsciously talking yourself out of them?

Creating New Thoughts

Begin by listening to every little thought, day dream, or fantasy that you have—nothing is insignificant. When you find yourself making a negative statement or having a negative vision, explore why it may be happening.

Do you have irrational fears left over from childhood? If so, replace them with realistic goals. Suppose, for example, that your inner voice tells you to eat everything on your plate when you go to a restaurant—you paid for it, after all. A more positive dialogue might go something like this: "Most of what I'm paying for is convenience and ambiance. The actual cost of the food itself is relatively minor. I'm only going to eat what I want."

Here's another example. You might say to yourself, "I'm going to follow this program 100 percent or not at all." Wow, those are high expectations! Here's a more realistic thought: "I'd like to be perfect, but I'm human. Striving for perfection only sets me up for failure. Each of these changes helps, so I'm going to start with what I can do, and add extra steps when I'm ready."

BOTTOM LINE: Lose 20–30 pounds

Suppose that turning negative thoughts into positive ones allows you to exercise 30 minutes a day—exercise you might not be getting otherwise. All by itself, this could help you lose 20–30 pounds in a year. Positive thoughts make it easier to eat more healthful meals. Count on saving 100 calories calories at every meal or 300 calories at dinner.

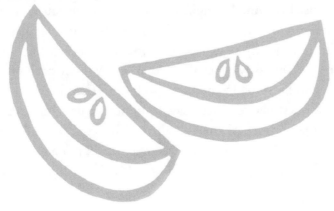

> **IF YOU** spend more than a few minutes on the phone at a time, you're probably wasting a golden opportunity to lose weight.

■ SOME telephone conversations require total concentration, but most are social chitchat. You can easily be doing something besides putting your feet up. My advice: Get that exercise bike spinning while catching up on your friends' latest dating fiascoes!

Even people who want to exercise don't always get around to it because it takes extra time. Well, here's the time. If the conversation is at all interesting, you'll probably forget that your legs are spinning beneath you.

It helps to get a cordless phone or even a headphone. And if you are going to be making a number of calls yourself, you might want to write the telephone numbers on Post-It notes and stick them on the bike. You can make all your calls without having to quit pedaling and look up a number!

BOTTOM LINE: Lose 10–42 pounds

Just how much weight can you lose while you're pedaling? Let's look at some numbers. Pedaling at 10 miles an hour (a relatively slow pace, easy to maintain while talking) for 25 minutes will burn 100 calories. A faster pace of 17 miles an hour for 15 minutes also burns 100 calories.

Modest phone talkers (say, 15 minutes a day) can lose up to 10 pounds a year this way. If you chat for 30 minutes to an hour daily, you could lose as much as 42 pounds.

Get spinning!

WHY would I suggest that you add something to your evening meal when you're trying to lose weight? Because salads are in a class by themselves.

■ GREEN salads are among the healthiest foods you can eat. They have almost no fat (assuming you don't drench them in full-fat Thousand Island). Just as important, they're high in fiber, which satisfies the appetite and makes you less likely to fill up on other, high-caloric foods. This is one reason I advise people to eat a salad at the beginning of a meal, not at the end.

I have nothing against iceberg lettuce, apart from the fact that it's low in fiber and virtually devoid of taste and texture. The best salads are made with other, more exciting greens, such as spinach, arugula, and so on. Throw in some vegetables for additional crunch, color, and flavor, as well as important nutrients.

Obviously, a salad is only as healthful as the topping. You'll definitely want to use a reduced-calorie dressing—and skip the fatty croutons, too.

Helpful: Put the dressing on the side of the plate or in a small bowl. Dip your fork in the dressing, then grab some greens. You'll get the same taste while limiting the calories.

BOTTOM LINE: Lose 36 pounds

I've found that people who enjoy a salad every lunch and dinner wind up saving about 320 calories a day, simply because they're eating less of other, more fattening foods.

REGRETTABLY, cooking oils and butter have the same amount of calories. Merely replacing one with the other won't help you lose weight—but you'll be a heck a of lot healthier.

■ BUTTER is full of saturated fat, the kind that clogs up your arteries. Oils, on the other hand, contain monounsaturated and polyunsaturated fats—the ones that help lower cholesterol and reduce the risk of heart disease. Olive, canola, and nut oils are among the best choices.

What about margarine? Nope. It's full of trans fats, which are just as bad for your heart as the saturated fat in butter. However, there are a few brands of margarine that contain no saturated or trans fats. These are acceptable.

Even though I started out by saying you can't lose weight by switching from butter to oils, that's not entirely true. If you give up butter entirely and use full-flavored oils in moderation, you'll find yourself cutting out quite a few calories.

Rather than smearing bread with butter, for example, dip it lightly in a dish of measured out olive oil. Sprinkle on some pepper or salt, if you like. The flavor goes a long way, so you don't have to use very much at all.

BOTTOM LINE: Lose 12 pounds

If switching from butter to oil causes you to use less fat—say, one less tablespoon a day—you could potentially lose up to 12 pounds a year.

I OFTEN explain to my clients that eating too quickly contributes to weight gain. But they still have trouble slowing down, so it's probably worth repeating.

■ SOME STUDIES indicate that it takes at least 20 minutes for your brain to get the signal that you've had enough to eat. Let's assume that you gobble down a complete meal in 10 minutes. Your brain won't realize that you've had enough to eat—or, more likely, that you're stuffed—until it's too late.

I'm not a big believer in that ancient advice that advocates chewing each bite 20, 30, or even 40 times. That's a little fussy for my taste. Just try to slow down.

How can you tell if you're eating too quickly? Well, if you often find yourself feeling uncomfortably full when you leave the table, that's a good sign. It means you're putting more food in your stomach than it needs—and you're doing it so quickly that your brain doesn't have time to respond.

Next time, take the time to enjoy and savor each bite. Start by taking a few deep breaths and relaxing before eating. You may want to put your fork down between bites. Chew the food thoroughly (without counting), swallow it, and relax for a moment. Then pick up your fork again.

BOTTOM LINE: Lose 10 pounds

People who eat more slowly invariably eat a little less. Every time you use this method at dinner, you can count on saving at least 100 calories.

#12 *hold the tuna salad*

MILLIONS of dieters think of tuna salad as the ultimate lean food that will help them lose weight. Bad news: It doesn't work.

■ IN FACT, you're probably better off eating a lean roast beef sandwich. Virtually every tuna salad you get in a deli or restaurant is prepared with lots of high-fat and high-calorie mayonnaise—and I mean *high!* The tuna was probably packed in oil. A sandwich made with turkey breast or lean roast beef, and without mayo, will dish up 200 fewer calories.

If you're making your own tuna salad, of course, you can enjoy tuna and cut the calories at the same time. If you substitute lite mayo for the full-fat kind, you'll save 100 calories. Or just use less regular mayo. Using water-packed tuna instead of oil-packed will save you another 100 calories.

The other advantage of homemade is that you can add all the fixings you really enjoy, such as pickles, onions, celery, carrots, capers, or even curry powder. The more highly seasoned ingredients you use, the less you'll notice the "missing" fat and calories.

BOTTOM LINE: Lose 3–6 pounds

Let's assume that you eat a tuna salad once a week. Substituting a homemade tuna salad or a turkey breast or lean roast beef sandwich will save you about 10,400 calories over the course of a year. If you're a real tuna lover who eats it more often, these simple substitutions can add up to some impressive weight loss!

TO BE FAIR, food pushers aren't bad people at heart. Your mom, your spouse, your friends—they just want to please you. But you have to be firm.

■ WE ALL know people who aren't satisfied until they convince us—*beg* us—to eat more, more, more. Their misguided entreaties are hard to resist, if only because we want to be polite.

The challenge is to say no in ways that work. After all, the food pusher is convinced that he or she is looking after your best interests.

I advise my clients to take a positive approach. Sample the proffered food, but tell your host, "This is delicious. I'd love to have more, but I'm totally full and can't take another bite." Positive, yet firm.

No matter what, don't hide behind the excuse that you're on a diet. This fails in three ways: (1) it gives the food pusher a double signal—that you really want it, but feel that you have to refuse; (2) it challenges the pusher to seduce you; and (3) it is sometimes taken as an insult, as though you're saying that the food isn't good enough for your refined tastes.

BOTTOM LINE: Lose 7 pounds

If you manage to resist a food pusher once a week, and decide not to have that 500-calorie dessert, you can easily lose 7 pounds in a year. The pushier your friends, the more weight you'll lose!

#14 *choose "surf"*

> **NEARLY** every restaurant offers a "surf" or "turf" special, or a combination of the two. Guess which one I recommend?

■ THE NUMBERS tell the story:

- 6-ounce slab of prime rib: 600 calories.
- 6-ounce sirloin: 450 calories.
- 6-ounce salmon: 400 calories.
- 6-ounce tuna steak: 250 to 300 calories.

Even though these are among the fattiest fish imaginable, they still have a lot fewer calories than red meat. They're also loaded with omega-3 fatty acids, which are good for your health, unlike the artery-clogging saturated fat in meat.

Stick with seafood as much as possible. A restaurant meal will always end up being richer than a meal at home, so it's worth cutting calories where you can. This means avoiding fried fish, of course; even blackened can be greasy. Stick to grilled, poached, or steamed fish.

BOTTOM LINE: Lose 4–18 pounds

Choosing salmon over prime rib could save 200 calories; a leaner fish (snapper, for example) will save you even more. For those hard-core meat eaters, switching to fish 6 out of 7 days can result in a weight loss of 18 pounds.

ACTUALLY, you have to tighten more than one, but that's the whole point: A technique called progressive relaxation has been proven to lower stress—and that, of course, lowers calorie intake at the same time.

■ THIS EASY procedure is among the best ways to lower physical and emotional stress. It relaxes your muscles and reduces your pulse rate, blood pressure, perspiration, and breathing rate. It physically relaxes your entire body, and people who do it regularly experience less of the negative side effects of stress overall.

We've already talked about the ways in which stress contributes to weight gain. Let's face it, we live in world where stress is omnipresent. Unfortunately, food is equally abundant. Put the two together, and you're going to see a lot of eating that has more to do with frustration and anxiety than with actual physical hunger.

It's not a coincidence that we all tend to gain weight during those times when life is most stressful—during transitions at work, for example, or in the course of divorces or other difficult life events, particularly events we can't contral. "Comfort food" makes us feel better temporarily, but the consequences can stick around for years.

Even if the stress in your life hasn't risen off the charts, all sorts of "negative" emotions—boredom, for example—promote the kind of mindless eating that quickly packs on the pounds.

I often recommend progressive relaxation for those with "type A" personalities. They tend to get bored with inactive forms of stress reduction, such as deep breathing (they respond, "Yeah, right!"). With progressive relaxation, you're actively tensing and relaxing the muscles, so it feels as though something is actually happening. Which, in fact, it is.

How to Do It

Progressive relaxation is a technique in which you tense, then relax, every muscle in your body, starting at the very tips of the toes and working all the way up to the head.

People generally find that it's easier to practice this technique when they're lying down, but you don't have to. Once you get good at it, you can practice it when you're sitting or even standing.

The muscle groups you want to work include the feet, legs, buttocks, abdomen, lower back, chest, shoulders, neck, face, and forehead.

Tense each group of muscles for about five seconds. Relax for a moment, take a breath, then move on to the next muscle group. Make sure your breathing is slow and steady throughout.

Mmmmm—it feels good! And you'll like the way you feel afterward, too.

BOTTOM LINE: Lose 19 pounds

Some people find that doing progressive relaxation daily makes it much easier to avoid afternoon or nightly snacks. Think about it: Passing on just one plate of nachos could save you 1,300 calories! So would avoiding your 185-calorie nightly snack.

> I DEFINE temptation as pushing a shopping cart down the ice cream aisle when you haven't eaten for 6 hours.

■ THINK of supermarkets as goodie factories for adults. When you're trying to lose weight, nothing is more hazardous than shopping when you're hungry. Foods that would never catch your eye when you're in your right mind will suddenly look very appealing.

I've witnessed this first hand. If I haven't eaten before I go shopping, I find myself tasting every piping-hot sample that's offered. Even the checkout line isn't safe. Some wicked candy bar is sure to leap off the shelf and into the pile of groceries. I suspect that they have Mexican jumping beans in them just for this purpose!

It's hard to say exactly how much of a difference eating before shopping will make. One of my clients, Lisa, said she probably consumed more than 300 calories in free tastings when she shopped on an empty stomach. Another client would get cravings—and buy all the ingredients for— coconut cake. Yet another routinely polished off bags of chips before she checked out.

Do yourself a favor. Eat, then shop.

BOTTOM LINE: Lose 9 pounds

My guess is that if you go shopping twice a week, and if you manage to eat before leaving home, you can count on saving yourself at least 300 calories each trip.

> **REGULAR** ice cream has **350** calories per cup.
> Fancy ice cream weighs in at **500** calories per cup.
> So quit eating ice cream already!

■ SORRY, I don't mean to sound harsh. But there are so many delicious desserts out there that won't blow your entire day's diet in a single shot. You don't have to have ice cream.

Try this instead. Buy some sweet cherries. Remove the pits and stems, and top them with a nice spoonful of whipped cream. It's delicious, and it's about as low-cal as you can ask for.

Let's take a look at the cherries. A quarter pound has 80 calories. A quarter cup of whipped cream—the pressurized kind you spray out of a can—has about 40 calories. Total caloric load: 120 calories. Compare that to the ice cream I mentioned earlier—or to whatever other sinful richness you have in mind—and the logic is inescapable.

I'm not insisting on cherries, by the way. Maybe your fruit of choice is a juicy pear. A crisp autumn apple. A bowl of berries. Have any of them. Have them all!

BOTTOM LINE: Lose 3–16 pounds

Depending on how often you make this switch, you can make significant strides in your weight loss. Suppose that you eat cherries and whipped cream instead of your usual ice cream once a week. That alone will account for 3–6 pounds of weight loss. Make the switch more often and you'll lose even more.

FORGET any lingering impressions of Eastern mysticism. Yoga today is as American as apple pie—and a lot healthier.

■ A FEW years ago, yoga seemed pretty exotic. Guys with long beards practiced yoga. College students with lava lamps and beads were into yoga. If my memory serves, the Beatles practiced yoga. Sure, it was good exercise, but it just seemed so—weird.

Hey, things have changed. Yoga has entered the American mainstream, and you'll find classes at YMCAs, community centers, and neighborhood recreation centers. Kids do yoga at school. Grandmothers do it at senior centers. Yoga is truly everywhere.

Yoga does have a long and complex tradition of mystical teachings, but that's not the way it's usually taught today. The yoga you're likely to encounter will consist of simple, gentle movements and stretching combined with deep diaphragmatic breathing. The exercises provide quite a workout, and the deep breathing is actually a form of meditation.

There's no question that yoga is one of the best forms of stress control—and, as I keep saying throughout this book, controlling stress is one of the best way to control appetite and weight gain.

If the idea of controlling stress and losing weight isn't enough to get you to sign up for a yoga class, here are some of the other benefits. It increases muscle and joint flexibility and strength. It improves range of motion and digestion. It helps relieve back pain and headaches. It can even lower blood pressure in some people.

My Story

I wasn't very successful when I tried to learn relaxation techniques. I was uptight to begin with, and I always found my mind going a mile a minute when I was supposed to be "mindlessly" communing with the universe. Oh, and I was a total failure at diaphragmatic breathing. I was raised by a military man, whose mantra was, "Stomach in, chest out"— the opposite of diaphragmatic breathing.

Nothing worked until I tried yoga. And then it clicked. Ever since, yoga has been one of the greatest discoveries of my life. After a session of yoga, I find myself more even tempered, rational, thoughtful, confident, and in control—of my life as well as my eating.

Anyone can perform yoga because the movements can be personalized to individual needs and limits. You can do it sitting, standing, or lying down. You can practice it for 15 minutes or two hours. It's all up to you.

BOTTOM LINE: Lose 13 pounds

Let's assume that you do a 15-minute yoga routine every evening. It's very likely to help you avoid your usual snacks of pretzels or whatever—and that can save you about 150 calories a night, 6 out of 7 nights.

■ **I'M TALKING** about salad, of course. Forget those creamy dressings. Go with vinaigrette: It's easy to make (or buy) and it has only a fraction of the calories.

■ THE MAIN reason I tell people to switch to oil-and-vinegar-based dressings is that they contain very little of the saturated fat that's found in traditional blue cheese or other creamy dressings. Saturated fat is the stuff that's converted into cholesterol in the blood and increases the risk of heart disease and stroke.

To be entirely honest, you won't save an amazing amount of calories when you switch to vinaigrettes—but you will save some. Blue cheese or creamy dressing has 60–80 calories per tablespoon, for example, compared to 50 in a vinaigrette, and about 40 in a "lite" reduced calorie vinaigrette.

Plus, vinaigrettes are wonderfully tangy and refreshing. You can buy them ready-made, but they're a snap to make at home: Try Dan Puzo's Vinaigrette on page 275. It's 45 calories per tablespoon and delicious! If you keep the vinaigrette in the refrigerator, it will stay fresh for more than a month.

BOTTOM LINE: Lose 13 pounds

Most people use at least four tablespoons of dressing on their salad. If you switch from a creamy dressing to vinaigrette, plan on saving 120 calories for every salad. Eat salads every day, and you could save 43,800 calories in a year!

> **LOSING weight is not about discipline or will-power. It's about controlling your environment. Period.**

■ WE ALL have different strengths and weakness, which must be considered when you're cutting calories or making any other healthful lifestyle changes.

Let's talk about me, Katherine Tallmadge. One of my main weaknesses is chocolate. I can't stop with one piece. That's simply not "normal" for me. I'll occasionally indulge my passion with a Dove bar or a piece of chocolate, but I've learned *never* to bring home a full box. It will be gone in a day or two, max.

I'm no better with chips. I have no self-control, and I know it. So I'll occasionally buy a 1-ounce bag. But a big bag? Never!

One of my strengths (finally, something positive!) is that I love fruits and vegetables. I stock up on these all the time.

You have to recognize your own "mines." I advise everyone to minesweep the kitchen for those calorie bombs that can explode your weight. Have a hard time resisting ice cream? Then get rid of the half-gallon. Candy bars your pitfall? Toss out the leftover bags from Halloween.

BOTTOM LINE: Lose 10–29 pounds

Minesweeping your kitchen periodically to get rid of things you shouldn't have in the house in the first place will save a tremendous amount of calories over time. Add the things that you like and should be eating, and you'll do even better.

> **NEARLY everyone loves a good, juicy hamburger. Are you one of them? No problem.**

■ HAMBURGERS are almost an institution in this country. I'm not one to criticize food choices (within reason), but the national fixation on hamburgers—and the frequency with which we enjoy them—definitely ranks among the main causes of weight gain.

Take Harry. One of my clients, he was all but addicted to burgers. He ate them for lunch at least twice a week, and burger dinners weren't unusual. Since the meat used in hamburgers ranges from fatty to fattier, he found himself getting a burger tummy.

No, I didn't advise Harry to quit eating hamburgers. He liked them too much, and I knew that a total prohibition would be counterproductive. All-or-nothing approaches, I've found, generally result in "nothing."

We came up with a more realistic plan. Harry was permitted—no, encouraged—to have burgers periodically, say, once a week. The rest of the time, he had to find other sandwiches that he enjoyed, but were much less likely to add inches to his waist.

Leaner Choices

What's a good burger substitute? Check out the deli department at the supermarket. You'll find all sorts of sandwich fixings that are full flavored as well as lean. To put this in perspective, half a pound of grilled hamburger meat has about 800 calories. The same amount of lean roast beef has half this amount.

Grilled chicken breast is an even better choice, with about 280 calories in half a pound. By substituting chicken for hamburger, you'll save 520 calories.

Of course, I'm only counting the calories in the meats themselves. Because switching to lean means results in such dramatic calorie reductions, you can be liberal in your choices of toppings. Want mayonnaise? Why not? A tablespoon of regular mayonnaise has 100 calories. You've saved so many calories by switching meats, you can afford the extra pleasure. Low-fat mayo has about half as many calories as regular. But by making the meat substitute, I can enjoy regular mayo without guilt.

Most sandwich add-ons don't have enough calories to worry about. Go ahead and load your sandwich with onion, lettuce, tomato, whatever you like. Just to keep it healthy, put it all between slices of whole-grain bread rather than the traditional white kind.

BOTTOM LINE: Lose 6–16 pounds

If you're in the habit of eating a hamburger or cheeseburger every week, and you make one of these meat substitutions weekly, you'll save enough calories over a year to drop six to eight pounds. Serious hamburger hounds who make the switch 3 times a week will lose a whole lot more.

> **EXERCISE can be a solitary affair, and some people get too bored to keep it up. So make it a group affair—and make yourself the center of the group.**

■ MY FRIEND Walsh joined an aerobics class full of women. He's the only man, which means he gets a lot of attention and reinforcement.

My mother began exercising for the first time in her life when a women-only gym opened in her area. She feels more comfortable when there aren't men around, and she gets a lot of attention from the trainers. She feels special at the gym, which is why she keeps going back.

I like company, too. Every Saturday, I take a walk with my good friend Tito. I look forward to these 5-mile walks through Rock Creek Park, and I go regardless of the weather. Walking with a friend makes the time go by pleasantly; it's sort of like a date, but without the romantic complications.

Speaking of romance, walking, rather than eating, is a great way to get to know someone. This is how I got to know Jack, my significant other. Talk about feeling special!

BOTTOM LINE: Lose 12 pounds

People who get extra attention when they exercise are more likely to keep it up. Let's assume, conservatively, that these good feelings motivate you to exercise 2 hours a week. You could lose as much as 12 pounds in a year!

#23 *the dilution solution*

> **HAVE** you noticed how big the soft drinks at convenience stores have gotten? Apart from the inevitable bathroom consequences, there's a huge amount of calories in those paper cups.

■ LINDA, a good friend, discovered this the hard way. Every day on her way to work, she would stop at the corner convenience store and tank up with a 32-ounce soda. She likes cold beverages, and she definitely likes caffeine. What she didn't appreciate, in retrospect, was the additional pounds she was putting on.

I'm always telling people to drink more water because it takes up room in the stomach and helps control appetite. It also has a lot fewer calories (none, actually) than sodas or other sweet beverages. Linda wasn't about to give up sodas, but she figured there had to be a way to get more water into the equation.

Here's what she started doing: Every time she bought a soda, she would cram the cup with ice, as much as it would hold. She figured that by the time the ice melted, she was drinking at least as much water as soda. Psychologically, however, she was satisfied because her morning ritual didn't change.

That's what I call creative thinking!

BOTTOM LINE: Lose 18 pounds

Let's assume that Linda cut her soda intake in half. That would mean that she was consuming 240 fewer calories every day she went to the office. That's better than you'll do by swearing off some sweet desserts!

THEY look healthy. They even taste healthy. But commercial muffins are little more than concentrated fat.

■ ARE you sitting down? Good, because the numbers I'm about to recite will take your breath away. Just one plump muffin—the super-sized kind sold today at supermarkets bakeries, and take-out shops—can set you back 600 calories. Eat one every day, and you'll consume about 219,000 calories a year. Yikes!

Low-fat muffins are much better. Even though a large one contains about 400 calories, that's a 200-calorie savings over the regular ones. I know, they don't taste quite as rich, but since you're eating them on the run anyway, you'll probably never notice!

Okay, you noticed. Why not make the muffin better by eating it with fruit? You can still do it on the run as long as you use whole fruit: take a bite of muffin, bite of fruit, bite of muffin....

Eventually, of course, you may want to give up the muffin altogether. It's a very high-calorie snack. That's a good idea. Even a low-fat muffin can put on some pounds, but fruit has no calories worth worrying about, and it's loaded with fiber and other important nutrients.

BOTTOM LINE: Lose 21–52 pounds

Switch from a fatty muffin to a low-fat muffin every day, and you can count on losing more than 20 pounds in a year. Give up muffins and switch to fruit, and you'll lose a lot— and I mean a lot—more.

ONE of my clients thought he was making dietary progress by switching from butter to margarine. Fact: All he was doing was swapping a batch of unhealthy manufactured chemicals for natural chemicals. He certainly wasn't losing weight.

■ BUTTER, except in small amounts as an occasional treat, is among the unhealthiest ingredients in the kitchen. Most margarine isn't any better, and even cooking oils, which have little saturated fat, are essentially concentrated calories.

You can't cook without oil of some kind. Butter and other oils sear the surfaces of foods and lock in juices and flavors. They also prevent sticking.

Fortunately, there is a compromise: vegetable oil spray.

Oil sprays such as Pam take the place of butter, margarine, and cooking oils when you're sautéing or frying foods. But because they're in a spray form, you're able to control with great precision the amount that goes in the pan. If you use pans with nonstick coatings, all it takes is a quick spritz.

I admit, oil spray doesn't lend foods anywhere near the same richness that you get with butter or margarine. But if you're using fresh, full-flavored ingredients to begin with, who needs the extra flavor?

BOTTOM LINE: Lose 10–31 pounds

Each tablespoon of butter or margarine has 100 calories. Substitute a vegetable oil spray for one tablespoon, and you could lose as much as 10 pounds a year. The more you substitute, the more you lose!

ONLY 7 PERCENT of Americans get the recommended kinds or amounts of disease-preventing, health-giving grains. Make sure you're in that 7 percent!

■ I ALWAYS advise people to choose foods that are made with whole grains, rather than refined grains such as white flour. Whole grains contain essential basic nutrients, along with antioxidants that help prevent disease.

Whole grains are probably the best single source of fiber. Fiber promotes weight loss by making you feel full on fewer calories. A high-fiber breakfast is almost guaranteed to curtail your hunger throughout the day.

The antioxidants in whole grains work together with fiber and other compounds to lower your risk for cancers and heart disease—by 30 to 40 percent, in some cases. In addition, the fiber in grains contributes to digestive health by keeping you regular.

Convinced? Good! Now, here's some advice. When buying bread, pasta, cereals, or even crackers, check the ingredients on the nutrition label. Whole wheat, whole oats, or whole something-or-other should be listed first. Use brown basmati rice or wild rice to increase your fiber. And look for bulgur—it's simply broken up whole wheat, and it's loaded with fiber. Use it instead of couscous or white rice, which have little nutritional value.

BOTTOM LINE: Lose 21 pounds

If you eat a serving of whole grain at each meal, and if it keeps you from eating an extra slice of bread or that extra half cup of pasta, you'll save 100 calories at lunch and dinner—that's 200 calories a day!

DID you know that Native Americans taught the Pilgrims how to prepare a slice of flame-seared pizza on an oyster shell—and that's why the Pilgrims praised God on the first Thanksgiving?

■ OKAY, enough silly historical revisionism. You get my drift. You can't get more American than pizza. And you can't get much healthier food, as long as you exercise some control over your choices.

Two slices of a cheese-only pizza from Domino's, assuming it's the 12-inch variety, will set you back 375 calories. An entire cheese pizza—small, with a thin crust—has 1,100 calories.

Even better are the frozen pizzas you make at home, either in the oven or in the microwave. (I recommend oven-baked because it has a crispier crust, and only takes a few minutes longer.) Check the calories on the box. Changes are, they'll total about 600. Even if you eat the whole thing yourself, you're getting a reasonably healthy meal.

Let's forget weight loss for a minute and talk about pizza sauce. All of those tomatoes in the sauce are loaded with lycopene, an antioxidant nutrient that has been shown to reduce the risk of prostate cancer in men. And since most men classify pizza as one of the main food groups, they're getting excellent protection!

BOTTOM LINE: Lose 3–6 pounds

Pretend it's Friday night and you're enjoying a homemade pizza or frozen instead of the usual greasy carryout. You'll save anywhere from 200–400 calories!

I'LL never forget those tomatoes. They were soft, plump, sweet, and deep red—the kind you only get fresh from the vine.

■ ONE of my favorite childhood memories is the taste of my grandmother's vine-ripened tomatoes. Every year, she grew at least 20 tomato plants—and only tomatoes—in her backyard in Columbus, Ohio. They were her favorite vegetable, and they became mine too.

It's funny how childhood experiences stay with us. Today, when I shop at a nearby farmers' market, I still revel in those feelings. Physically I am in downtown Washington, D.C., but mentally and emotionally I am picking my grandmother's tomatoes in Columbus!

Enough nostalgia. In my practice, I often instruct clients to visit farmers' markets in their neighborhoods. This has nothing to do with warm and fuzzy; it's because I've found that they lose weight even when they don't make any other changes.

Here's what happens. You go to the farmers' market and stock up on beautiful produce. The more fresh and delicious produce you eat, the less junk you consume, and the more weight you lose.

BOTTOM LINE: Lose 36 pounds

Fresh produce from a farmers' market will make you hungry for a salad every day. Adding salads to your daily meals will help you cut back on other, more fattening foods. Those delicious fresh fruits do the same thing. You'll lose an impressive amount of weight—and that's without dieting!

> **ONE** of my friends, Debbie, was furious when she discovered that her television had been stolen when she was on vacation. But a few weeks later came the unexpected surprise: She was losing weight.

■ I'VE heard variations of this story before, and it makes a certain amount of sense. Watching television doesn't require a tremendous amount of concentration, so we often do other things at the same time—eating being one of the main ones.

Most of us enjoy nibbling chips, popcorn, candies, or other snacks while we're watching TV. Because our minds are on the television, we're not really paying attention to how our bodies are feeling, which means we often consume more calories than we need.

Try something creative. Make a pact with a friend: "I'll 'steal' your TV if you 'steal' mine. We'll donate both of the 'stolen' TVs to Goodwill."

Once the TV is out of the house or in a "TV room" away from where you eat, you'll almost automatically snack less. Plus, think about all the free time you'll have. You won't have any choice but to find more creative things to do, and the more creative and busy you are, the less vulnerable you'll be to food cravings.

BOTTOM LINE: Lose 27 pounds

I sometimes advise people to think of TV as the equivalent of having a 19-inch brownie in the house. If you give it up, you're going to give up calories at the same time—probably about 300 a night.

BAGGY clothes get more and more attractive when you've gained extra weight. They're comfortable, and they also hide what's happening with your body. Can you say "denial"?

■ NEARLY everyone I know has a closetful of out-sized clothing—skirts, blouses, and pants that are a few sizes larger than they used to be. I understand the temptation to let out your clothes or buy larger sizes when you've gained extra weight, but it's the wrong thing to do.

It's all about psychology. "Fat" clothes can make you feel fat. They're also a sign that you've accepted being heavy.

Do just the opposite. Even when you're home alone, wear clothes that fit well. Forget the baggy robe or sweat pants. Wear a form-fitting leotard or fitted pants. You'll feel good when you wear good clothes, you'll also be reminded to think slim, and you'll be less likely to overeat if it feels uncomfortable or worse—if it shows! Any reminder to consume fewer calories can be helpful when you're trying to shed pounds.

BOTTOM LINE: Lose 9 pounds

Suppose that wearing fitting clothes around the house reminds you of your long-term fitness goals and keeps you from eating from a 300-calorie snack on the weekends. You're going to lose weight!

> **ONE of my clients, Sally, loves hearts of palm. She rarely buys those little cans, however, because they're frighteningly expensive. Then she had a revelation.**

■ HEARTS of palm are very low in calories. True, a single can may cost more than a full meal, but Sally figured that the high cost would be more than offset by the calorie savings.

Here's what she did. She started buying hearts of palm and keeping them on her shelf. Why? Because she loves adding them to salads. She realized that if she could enjoy hearts of palm every night, she would eat salads every night, and that in turn would help her control her weight. That's good value for the money!

Maybe you have a passion for shrimp, kiwi fruit, or crab meat. Don't worry about the cost (remember, you're not using huge amounts). Think about all of the delicious, nutritious meals you'll be able to make. If having a special food in the house helps you eat more of the foods you know are good for you, the cost is justified.

And the cost, incidentally, will be lower than you think. When you're eating more healthful foods, you'll naturally buy fewer junk foods, and when you're at a healthy weight, you have *half* the medical costs. So you'll actually be *saving* money.

BOTTOM LINE: Lose 17 pounds

I mentioned earlier that adding a salad to your lunch and dinner can save you 320 calories. If adding your favorite delicacy helps you eat one of those salads, you could lose 17 pounds!

YOU probably have a hobby that you'd like to take up, but can never find the time. Well, make the time! Hobbies are a lot of fun, and they can help you lose weight.

■ SEWING gives me great pleasure. I do it in the evenings after work, and it helps me forget about the day's frustrations and worries. Plus, I get to create beautiful things I can wear. What could be better for a clotheshorse like me?

I regularly take classes from an expert sewer. This past year, I learned how to make perfectly fitting pants for the first time. I now have three basic pants patterns: pleated baggy pants, flat front straight-legged pants, and casual drawstring pants, all in a variety of fabrics.

Sewing is obviously my thing. What's yours? You may enjoy making window treatments, place settings, or holiday presents. Maybe you've always thought about collecting coins, painting, or playing the piano. My friend Lind started piano lessons at age 40, and it's enriched her life.

Hobbies are a wonderful way to relax and unwind. They keep your mind and hands busy—and out of the pantry or refrigerator all of those times when you're feeling tired or a little bored.

BOTTOM LINE: Lose 9 pounds

I've never done the math, but I suspect that my hobby has saved me hundreds of thousands of calories over the years. I figure that if I sew 2 evenings a week, and avoid the snacks I would have had otherwise, I can save 600 calories.

HAVE you noticed that the sounds of work have gotten louder? Instead of the whisking of a rake, we're bombarded with the blast of leaf blowers. When's the last time you heard the tsk-tsk of a push mower? Sure, power tools are easy to use—and that's precisely the problem.

■ A QUICK equation: If you clear your yard with a leaf blower, you'll burn about 4 calories a minute. Use a rake, you'll burn 6 calories. Doesn't sound like much? Well, consider this.

Jobs done with traditional tools take longer than those done with power tools. This means you're going to get more exercise no matter what. Let's assume that you mow your lawn 10 times during the summer (and have to remove the clippings), and you rake leaves twice during the fall. I don't know how big your yard is, but we'll further assume that your total calorie expenditure with the leaf blower is about 60, while plying the rake burns 80 calories.

Guess what? That's enough to lose a pound right there. If you have a lot of trees, a wide expanse of grass, and you're particular about the way your yard looks, you're going to lose impressive amounts of weight.

BOTTOM LINE: Lose 5 pounds

Hand tools don't require gas or much in the way of maintenance, and they're great for your health. And they're a heck of a lot quieter than power tools, which will make your neighbors very happy! Lose 5 pounds for every season yopu rake by hand.

MANY health and political organizations sponsor marches to raise money as well as awareness. It's a chance to make your voice heard—and get some exercise at the same time.

■ A CLIENT of mine lost her mother to breast cancer, and decided to get involved. To honor her mother and help raise money for breast cancer research, she signed up for a 3-day, 60-mile walk.

Walking 60 miles, if you haven't done it lately, is a heck of a lot of exercise. At the very least, it requires a few weeks (and preferably months) of training. And that's what my client Renee did. She took a lot of shorter walks in order to get in shape for the big event. By the time the march rolled around, she had already lost 30 pounds.

Since then, she has gotten involved in a number of other causes, and marching has become her way of speaking out. She appreciates the exercise, especially because she's helping herself and others at the same time. As a bonus, getting involved in causes has increased her sense of confidence and self-worth, and this in turn has encouraged her to lose weight and look her best.

BOTTOM LINE: Lose 60 pounds

Getting involved in community and national causes is a great way to pump extra meaning into your life. And if you walk 40–50 miles a week, you can expect to lose about 60 pounds.

> **LUNCH** should supply important nutrients, be reasonably low in calories, and keep your energy high all afternoon. The humble sandwich does all three.

■ I LOVE sandwiches, salads, and soups for lunch. I feel particularly good, and am most productive, on afternoons when I haven't overeaten. At the same time, I need to eat enough so that I won't have cravings a few hours later.

The easiest way to meet these goals is to make a sandwich—assuming, of course, you have the fixings on hand. The next time you go shopping, pick up a loaf of whole wheat bread, a jar of mayonnaise ("lite," if you prefer), sliced, reduced-fat cheese, and several luncheon meats. Today's stores have lean versions of everything: lean bologna, turkey bologna, extra-lean ham—all kinds of lean. I've found that half a pound of cheese and a pound and a half of luncheon meats is enough to make a sandwich every day of the week.

A good sandwich also needs produce. I might buy 14 tomatoes at the farmers' market, so I can have 2 tomatoes each day for lunch. I'll also pick up bags of greens for green salads. (Out of season, I buy greens at the grocery store.) For salad dressing, I'll buy a bottle of "lite" whatever, or I'll make my own vinaigrette at home.

BOTTOM LINE: Lose 21 pounds

When I have all the necessary ingredients and prepare my own lunch, it saves me at least 200 calories daily. As an added bonus, I feel alert all afternoon because I haven't overeaten.

> **NO ONE** believes me when I tell them that they can burn 600 calories before going to work or before even waking up! They look even more surprised when I explain that it's the best way to do it.

■ EVERYONE knows they should exercise. Some people even want to exercise. But it's virtually impossible to do once you've embarked on the daily routine of carpooling children, getting through the workday, or running from class to class. Let's be honest: Even on those days when you plan to exercise, you'll often find a way to cancel it.

Try this: Wake up in the morning. Yawn. Roll out of bed, go to the bathroom, have a drink of water, and slip on some exercise clothes. Don't check e-mail or phone messages. Start moving. Now! Right away! Exercising first thing in the morning is one of the best things you'll ever do for yourself. And before you know it, it's over with before you're even awake!

Here are some of the reasons. (1) Showering after your exercise session will relax and awaken you at the same time. (2) Morning exercise is like taking an energy pill. You'll drink less coffee, which means your entire day will go better—and you won't experience that afternoon dip in your attention span. (3) You'll know that you've done it! Exercise is out of the way, so you don't have to wonder when you're going to fit it in. You'll be able to spend the rest of the day concentrating on all the other things you want to do.

A Success Story

Dan, one of my clients, is an adviser to corporations around the world. Once his day starts, he's at the mercy of his clients, who include secretaries of state and members of the president's cabinet. Dan loves his job. He loves it so much that he would much rather please his clients than take care of himself.

From long experience, Dan has learned that he *has* to exercise first thing in the morning. If he doesn't, it will never happen.

Without fail, he gets on a treadmill for 30 minutes every morning before he goes to the office. Three times a week, he meets with a personal trainer—early in the morning, of course.

Oh, one more thing. Dan did something radical in the business world: He adopted a no-breakfast-meetings policy. What has this intransigence cost him? Well, he's still in demand—and he's lost 20 pounds in the few months since he started!

BOTTOM LINE: Lose 28–42 pounds

All it takes is 30 minutes in the morning: Just walking briskly will burn up to 28 pounds in a year. Jogging on a treadmill will burn even more. Another great thing about morning exercise: You do it at the best time of day, without midday heat to contend with.

YOU CAN LOSE an amazing amount of weight just by having more fun in your life—especially when you're having that fun on company time.

■ LET ME TELL you about Jay. A computer whiz (and a client), Jay used to sit on his butt all day in front of his monitor. Largely because of his lack of activity for at least 8 hours a day, Jay found himself registering 250 pounds on the scale.

My solution: I advised Jay to become the founding member of the "Tour d'office." Every hour on the hour throughout the day, Jay starts a brisk, 5-minute walk down the office corridors. He invites everyone to follow him—and they wind through the halls doing a snake dance.

It's not the type of thing that *seems* like exercise, but it is—very good exercise, I might add. See if you can do something similar without interrupting work too much. Snake through the halls. Dance around the cafeteria or in the parking lot. Bring along a portable CD player and blast Caribbean rhythms to spur everyone on.

Other ideas: Take pictures of all the fun and post them on the office bulletin board; set up (non-food) rewards for the people who participate consistently; and get the boss involved (good luck!).

BOTTOM LINE: Lose 24 pounds

If you follow Jay's plan and move at a brisk pace, you'll find yourself burning about 8 calories per minute; 40 calories in 5 minutes; 320 calories each work day; and *83,000* calories a year!

#38 *buy better dairy*

MILK AND OTHER dairy foods are incredibly nutritious. Too bad they're also fattening—unless you choose wisely.

■ MANY of my clients won't touch dairy foods because they don't want the extra calories. I gently try to set them straight. Dairy products are by far the best source of calcium, the mineral that protects against osteoporosis.

Traditional dairy products are high in saturated fat. But things have changed. If your goal is to lose weight, there are many fantastic dairy products that will help you do it.

Suppose you switch from whole milk to 2%: you'll save 20 calories per serving. Switch from 2% to skim: another 20 calories saved. Low- or reduced-fat cheeses can save you 30 to 50 calories per ounce, depending on the type you buy. And substituting low-fat yogurt for whole yogurt saves at least 50 calories per cup.

Even if you are lactose-intolerant, you should be able to drink half a cup of milk 4 times a day without symptoms. Lactase-fortified milk can help. You can add lactase tablets to milk before drinking it. Or you can have milk, cheese, or yogurt made with soy, which doesn't cause discomfort.

Important: When buying soy products, check the label to make sure they're calcium fortified. Each serving should provide a third of the daily calcium requirement, just as dairy products do.

BOTTOM LINE: Lose 16 pounds

Substitute 3 daily servings of low-fat dairy food for the full-fat kind, and you'll cut out about 150 calories daily.

BELIEVE it or not, your feet should do more than keep a footstool company in front of the TV. In the primitive days of yore, they were actually used for locomotion!

■ AMERICANS don't walk very much anymore. We're also heavier than ever before. Hmm...I wonder if there's a connection?

Robert, one of my clients, is a case in point. He wasn't much of a walker, and he was having a heck of a time losing weight. Then the elevator at his office went on the blink. He started walking up the stairs out of necessity.

One thing led to another. He kept taking the stairs even when the elevator was repaired, and he walked at other times, as well. Did he lose weight? Yes—and he did it with almost no effort and without dieting.

To reacquaint yourself with your feet, you could follow Robert's example and use stairs instead of elevators. Or climb the stairs part of the way, then take the elevator the rest.

Another tip: When you drive to work, park at the far reaches of the parking lot and walk the rest of the way. It won't add up to heavy exercise, but it will make a difference.

BOTTOM LINE: Lose 11–22 pounds

Climbing stairs consumes, on average, 15 calories per minute. Let's say you do it for 10 minutes each work day. In a year's time you'll lose 11 pounds. Climb those same stairs for another 10 minutes at your lunch break and you'll lose at least twice that much. *In just minutes.*

> **BASIC KITCHEN TOOLS are important. But to lose weight, there's no substitute for good kitchen gadgets.**

■ I'M NOT TALKING about lemon zesters and in-the-shell egg beaters—those intriguing utensils that people buy, use once, then lose at the bottom of a kitchen drawer. I'm talking about gadgets that reduce fat consumption, control calories, and make batch cooking a dream.

What you *have* to have:

- Two nonstick 8" or 10" sauté pans. You'll use a lot less fat with nonstick coatings.
- 2-quart and 3-quart sauce pans.
- A heavy-duty stockpot—perfect for large batch recipes.
- A food scale to help you get a handle on proper serving sizes.
- Plastic containers that are freezer- and microwave-safe. Get large as well as portion-sized containers.
- Baggies for leftovers, cut-up fruits and vegetables, and for taking lunch to the office. Get pint, quart, and half-gallon sizes

BOTTOM LINE: Lose 12–52 pounds

If you make every recipe in nonstick utensils, and use one less tablespoon of oil a day, you'll save 120 calories—and lose up to 12 pounds—in a year. Packing a container with a healthy lunch will save you 400 calories a day, compared to what you'd consume if you splurged in a restaurant. That healthy fruit snack in a baggie? It has about 150 fewer calories than many high-fat snacks. As for portion control, count on saving 250 calories daily because you won't overestimate the amount you need to eat. We all tend to be overly generous to ourselves that way!

BEFORE you eat anything, take your food to the table. Sit down, close your eyes, and take three or four deep breaths to relax your mind and body.

■ DO THIS with *every* morsel of food you consume, whether it's a peanut or a slice of pot roast—or even the tasting that you do when you're cooking.

Hey, what's wrong with slowing down? I'm not suggesting "do not eat." All I'm saying is that you should take the time to sit down and really get to *know* that you are eating, and what you are eating.

Step back in time for a moment. When you were an infant, and later as a child, you knew when you were hungry, when you were not hungry, and when you were satisfied after being hungry. You ate and stopped eating appropriately in response to those signals. No matter how delicious a food was, or how much you loved it, if you weren't hungry, your mother could not get you to eat it. If you don't believe me, ask her!

As the years went by, you (along with every other human adult on the planet) began to eat in response to external signals. For example:

■ Time of day: "Hey, it's dinner time" or "You can't eat now, it's not time."

■ The presence of food: "Look at that delicious pie! Let's have some!"

■ Pleasing a loved one: "I made your favorite key lime pie, honey, have a piece."

■ Parental reinforcement: "If you're good, you'll get some caramels!"

■ Anger: "You can't have any, you've been bad!"

■ Feelings: "Have some ice cream, you'll feel better."

All of these are reasons for eating—and none have anything to do with hunger!

Learning to listen to your body's *real* hunger signals all over again is one of the keys to long-term weight maintenance. It takes practice and attention, but awareness is the first step. Once you master eating in response to your body's signals, your body will fall back into its natural healthy shape, and stay there forever.

BOTTOM LINE: Lose 17 pounds

One of my clients, Michael, is a big eater. When he started to practice "mindful" eating, he was amazed to discover that he was often perfectly content to leave food on his plate. In other words, he was satisfied with less than he was before.

If you eat out a lot in restaurants, where portions are extra large, mindful eating can make an impressive difference. If, for example, being deeply aware of your body and the food in front of you causes you to eat two fewer slices of bread than usual, you'll save 160 calories. That really adds up!

BET you never heard that before. But it's true: People who snack throughout the day find it easier to lose weight because they actually take in fewer calories.

■ "SNACK" is a loaded word. In our society, it has come to mean something "extra," or at least fattening. That's not the way to think of it. Snacks give you calories when you need them. Snacks keep you satisfied, so you're less likely to experience runaway hunger or emotional cravings.

Snacks have to be planned, of course. Otherwise, you'll find yourself stuck with whatever's available, even if that means foraging in your coworker's desk.

My favorite snack is fresh fruit. It gives you a sweet fix, and it makes you feel full, but not too full. If fruit alone doesn't satisfy your hunger, try garnishing it. Smear a tablespoon of peanut butter on your crunchy apple—yum! The peanut butter only adds 90 calories, and they are 90 satisfying and healthy calories. Or have a handful (a small one) of nuts along with the apple.

Other options: Have an ounce of cheese with your fruit. Or, if you're really hungry, some yogurt. Since midday snacks reduce the amount of lunch or dinner you'll need, don't worry about the few extra calories.

BOTTOM LINE: Lose 19–26 pounds

If your healthy snack keeps you from your usual vending machine pick-me-up, you'll save about 250 calories right there. Do it every day, and you'll lose a lot of weight in a hurry.

> **YOUR MOTHER, your hairdresser, and your shrink have all told you to get at least 8 hours of sleep a night. So why aren't you doing it—especially now that you're trying to lose weight? Maybe it's time to enlist the help of your VCR.**

■ I HAD NEVER thought about VCRs as a tool for weight loss until I talked to Robert, an unusually discerning client who had struggled for a long time to keep his weight under control.

At some point, Robert began to pay attention to his nightly routine. He discovered an interesting pattern. By 10 o'clock at night, he was usually yawning and ready for bed, yet he stayed up until after midnight. Why? Because he was a Letterman freak. He couldn't bear to hit the sheets until he'd laughed at David's latest stupid pet tricks.

Upon further reflection, Robert realized that these Letterman comedy routines would be just as funny the next day. That's when his dust-gathering VCR came to the rescue. He began setting the VCR to tape that night's show. Once the machine was set, Robert went to bed. The next evening, right after dinner, he'd relax by watching the previous night's show. By 9:30 he was ready to reset the VCR once again.

Robert's Inventory of Benefits

We still haven't talked about why using a VCR in general, or taping Letterman in particular, helped Robert lose weight. Here are some of the reasons:

■   Robert was now getting to bed early enough to pack in his eight hours of sleep. That made him more alert the next day—and the more alert he felt, the less likely he was to turn to snacks for "artificial" energy.

- Robert's late-night sessions with Letterman invariably involved munching. Getting his "late-night" TV fix right after dinner, when his stomach was already satisfied, meant fewer empty calories later on.

- Early to bed, early to rise. Robert found that he now had enough time in the mornings to exercise and eat a healthful breakfast. Big-time calorie savings, there.

- For some clients, THIS IS IT! If you get enough sleep, exercise 30 minutes in the morning, and eat a big breakfast, that's enough to lose all the weight you want and feel great forever. Just ask Vivien and Dan and Michael and Jay and . . . etc., etc.

BOTTOM LINE: Lose 16–66 pounds

Just cutting out late-night snacking saved Robert 150 calories a night. A healthy breakfast—and less snacking later—added up to more saved calories, and his newfound exercise routines also did their part.

To break it down, Robert stood to lose 16 pounds by not snacking at night; 20 pounds from the exercise, and another 30 pounds by preparing his own breakfast which prevented him from indulging in the 200-calorie midmorning doughnut and from attacking lunch and saving at least 100 calories there. Love that Letterman!

ACTUALLY, you don't have to go that far. But you should focus your entire attention on your food. Enjoy and savor every bite.

■ TOO OFTEN, our meals are overwhelmed by distractions. The TV in the background. Music on the stereo. The newspaper propped against a cereal box. Add internal distractions, such as work worries, and the food itself gets scant attention.

Why is this a problem? Because when you eat on autopilot, when your mind is somewhere else, you don't enjoy your food very much. More important, "mindless" eating generally turns into overeating. When eating doesn't provide psychological satisfaction, you'll crave more food than your body actually needs.

Eating a delicious meal deserves your entire attention. After all, you're feeding your body, and what's more important than that? So turn off the electronic gizmos. Think about what you're eating: the taste, texture, aroma, and so on. If you're dining with someone, put your fork down when you want to talk. Pick it up again when you're ready to pay attention to the food.

This is especially important at work. Get away from your desk if you can—and if you can't, at least don't talk on the phone or work while you eat.

BOTTOM LINE: Lose 21 pounds

Once you start focusing your attention on the food in front of you, you'll almost automatically eat a little less. In fact, even if you leave only a few extra bites on your plate, it could add up to a savings of 200 or more calories daily.

> WHEN we were infants, we couldn't wait to get off our knees and start walking. Now that we're adults, it's a different part of our bodies that we have to get off of.

■ DOES YOUR derriere get more of a workout than your legs? That's a real problem if you're trying to lose weight.

The solution (sigh of relief) isn't hard-core exercise. All you really have to do is get walking. Long, brisk walks are good, but so are strolls and ambles. Walking the dog. Going to the mailbox. *Any* kind of walking will help you burn calories and lose weight.

Where you walk is up to you, but make it someplace pleasant that will contribute to your motivation. If you have to drive to get to your starting point, at least that's putting the buggy to good use! You'll walk a lot more if the place you like to walk is easy to get to.

Helpful: Buy an inexpensive pedometer at a sporting goods store. You'll have an accurate record of how far you're walking, which is great for motivation. Wear comfortable walking shoes, as well as layers of clothing to take off as you get warm, or put back on when you're cooling off.

BOTTOM LINE: Lose 6–14 pounds

Walking briskly for 1 mile, 3 times a week, will add up to about 21,060 calories burned in a year. Do it every day, and you'll lose impressive amounts of weight in a hurry!

> **THE food diary is the main tool for self-examination of your eating habits.**

■ SOCRATES told us that the road to wisdom is to know ourselves. This is never more true than in your eating habits. So often we eat without thinking that we literally don't know what we are eating—or that we are eating.

It is important that you begin observing objectively what you eat and the way you eat, for this is the cornerstone of your program: your own observations.

That's what Frank discovered. Frank, a 39-year-old defense department employee, lost 2 pounds during a week in which he was simply keeping a diary. He swore he ate normally, just as usual—and even everything he wanted. The same thing happened with Deborah. She was shocked (pleasantly!) when she stepped on the scale and found she lost four pounds. While Miriam, a 50-year-old writer, found that keeping the diary helped stop her weight from spiraling upward, where it had been going for several weeks, if not months.

The reason: Just paying attention was enough to make a difference! The diary, called a self-monitoring device in behavior modification lingo, plays three important roles.

First, if it is kept at the time of eating or within 15 minutes, it can change behavior as behavior occurs—and without your even realizing it or trying to change. For instance, Ella, a wife, mother of 2 and government lawyer, found that she was consuming most of her day's calories—almost subconsciously—while cooking dinner. This was happening so automatically that she didn't even know she was doing it until she began writing it down. Of course, having to write down every little item while she was trying to cook became tiresome so her desire to eat decreased. Also, just the realization that she was, in effect, eating two dinners every night gave her impetus to change.

Debra C., on the other hand, found that without even thinking about it, she grabbed M&Ms from a coworker's candy bowl every time she walked by. This, of course, began adding up after the 8th or 10th time! And because of the way she was grabbing the candies on the go, she realized she wasn't even tasting or enjoying them. Her heightened awareness began to inhibit the behavior. Peter H. found he didn't even know he was eating or how much, since others always prepared his food—until he began observing, asking questions, and started seeing it written down in black and white.

The diary allows you to differentiate between unconscious eating and savoring what you really enjoy. All of these people are successes. They may not have been perfect—or have lost weight, but they kept the diary at the time of eating and learned about themselves and their eating habits. And what's especially telling is none of them realized they had made changes until we sat and talked while looking over their week's diary in detail. This is one of the beauties of keeping the diary uncritically; you begin to learn and then evolve on your own.

Research shows this way of changing is more likely to succeed long term: that is, observing your behaviors and making decisions about changes to make. And remember, I am simply your guide, helping you discover and learn, whereas you are the creator and owner of your own success...and you can make your dreams come true!

The second function of the food diary is simply learning. At the end of each day, week or month, you can look back and analyze for yourself what style of eating works for you.

This brings us to the third function of the diary, which is helping you individualize your weight loss program so that it fits into your lifestyle and is something you enjoy living with. Now, isn't this the only way to do things?

Individualizing your plan is critical to your long-term success because nothing can last unless it is enjoyable and works into your lifestyle. Through keeping the diary consistently, you can find that perfect "middle ground" for you. You will be able to eat in a way which you enjoy and can live with, but which also achieves your weight and health goals.

BOTTOM LINE: Lose 23 pounds

If keeping the diary enhances your attentiveness and helps you eat less here or there or even think twice about that vending machine candy bar, you could save 220 calories per day.

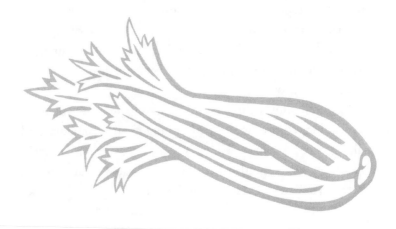

5

How to Beat Emotional Eating

Especially appropriate for: *Cravers, Bingers, Self-saboteurs, People who are "hungry all the time," Those who eat too fast or with too many distractions, Those who are out of touch with their feelings, Positive thinkers, Negative thinkers*

One of my clients, Ellen, complained that she felt hungry all the time. She couldn't control her eating—or lose the 10 pounds that she needed to lose to get back into her favorite clothes.

Gary had a different story. He craved sweets constantly, especially at the office. His doctor told him that he had to lose 30 pounds and lower his cholesterol.

Kelly, another client, told me that she felt out of control. She was bingeing all the time, and was seeing a psychotherapist. But her wedding was in a few months, and she wanted desperately to lose 20 pounds.

Catherine's story really hit home, mainly because it was so typical. She wanted to lose weight, and often she would. But then she'd find herself sabotaging her efforts.

Ellen, Gary, Kelly, and Catherine are all very different people, but with something in common: Their eating habits were a mess. They ate for reasons that had nothing to do with hunger. They didn't understand—or at least weren't able to put into practice—the most basic rules of feeding their bodies appropriately. My job was to help them unlearn the lousy lessons they had picked up from years of dieting.

Losing weight often has less to do with specific food choices than with the underlying emotions. People have a hard time understanding that their feelings, and the unconscious self-talk that we all listen to every day, play a critical role in eating decisions.

I've found that most people who have difficulty controlling their weight have never learned how to listen to their feelings or to their bodies. They don't always recognize when they're stressed, depressed, or frustrated, and they certainly don't recognize when they're using food as a way to cope.

My experience has taught me that most people with an "unhealthy" relationship to food, whether that involves out-of-control cravings or anything else, need first of all to understand the importance of careful meal planning and eating meals at regular times. Once their bodies fall into a natural rhythm, it's much easier for them to *feel* the difference—and to stick with the healthy changes.

Weight-related eating problems may seem complicated, but they're not. With sensitive and nonjudgmental self-exploration, nearly everyone can learn to eat normally and keep their weight under control.

HUNGER is pretty rational. It tells you when you need to eat and when you've had enough. Cravings, on the other hand, are cruel and capricious. They always demand more, more, more!

■ FOOD CRAVINGS are your enemy. They're the beasts inside you that can make it almost impossible to lose weight—unless you learn to put them in their place.

What's the difference between hunger and cravings? Hunger means your body is running low on energy. Think of it as the warning light that tells you when to eat. Cravings, on the other, live in your emotions. When you're frustrated, tense, tired, depressed, in love, out of love, or whatever, cravings push you toward food in an attempt to quiet the turbulence within.

People who are successful at losing weight have learned to distinguish true hunger from cravings. In other word, they listen to their stomachs, not their emotions.

The Hunger Test

Because we all eat for emotional reasons as well as for hunger, it's not always easy to tell them apart. The real difference between them becomes apparent after you're done eating. If hunger was in charge, you should feel pretty good—satisfied, but not stuffed. If cravings had the upper hand, well, reach for the Alka Seltzer!

When you give in to cravings, you are abusing your body, plain and simple. You are forcing your body to store excess calories as fat. You are also abusing a substance—food—by using it for something other than hunger.

My clients are amazed at how much less food they need in order to feel comfortable. Take Ann. She always ate two cups of pasta, even though she left the table feeling uncomfortably full. I convinced her to cut back to one cup, and guess what? She felt terrific, and not ready for a nap the way she had been in the past.

Using a scale of 0-10,* rate your body's hunger signals before you begin eating and when you finish:

  0 = Ravenous: Irrational...will eat anything
  1 = Empty: Too hungry, a bit irrational
  2 = Hungry: Time to eat
  3 = Hungry-or-Light: You could eat or you could wait
  4 = Light: You should wait before eating
  5 = Comfortable: You are no longer hungry, satisfied, comfortable without feeling full
  6 = Slightly Uncomfortable: Very subtly past comfort level
  7 = Uncomfortable
  8 = Full: Your waistband is tightening
  9 = Very Full: You're having to move your belt a notch
10 = Overstuffed

BOTTOM LINE: Lose 30 pounds

If listening to your body signals means you don't clean your plate automatically or eat for emotional reasons if you regularly eat when your stomach registers a "2," and stop eating when it registers a "5," count on saving at least 300 calories a day.

* Adapted from *Eating Awareness Training* by Molly Groger (Summit Books, 1983)

BELIEVE it or not, the biggest cause of food cravings and bingeing is undereating. Go too long
without food, and the body becomes ravenous—
and irrational.

■ YOUR BODY normally gets hungry every 3 to 5 hours,
depending on the size of your meals. Eating regularly during
the day gives you the most control over food cravings and
bingeing.

I usually advise people to eat 5 times a day: breakfast,
snack, lunch, snack, dinner. If you prefer just 3 meals, that
can work too, provided the meals are balanced, and your
breakfast, lunch, and dinner are roughly equal in calories.
For most people, that means switching some calorie intake
from dinner to breakfast.

This sort of regular routine maintains your body's normal hunger signals, the highest metabolic rate, and the most
efficient burning of calories. And, most important, it gives
you more control over your impulses.

Let's take a look at this. Impulse eating, or bingeing, is
usually a result of poor planning. In other words, you'll find
yourself in the wrong place (near a vending machine or a
fast-food restaurant) at the wrong time (when you're starving). If you eat at regular times and never let yourself get too
hungry, this is much less likely to occur.

Incidentally—and to repeat—I advise everyone to eat
dinner at least three hours before going to bed. Try to make
this the last time you eat because calories that are consumed
late are more likely to wind up as fat than calories consumed
earlier. Still, be flexible. It's fine to have a light snack—fruits

or vegetables are ideal—after dinner if you're hungry. Just be sure that you're not reaching for food for other reasons—because you're bored, for example, or because you're stressed about work or personal problems.

How does all of this add up to weight loss? Let's take a look:

- If you have a fruit snack at regularly scheduled times, you'll be less likely to raid the vending machine. That could add up to 20 lost pounds a year.
- Planning your meals ahead of time allows you to have nutritious homemade food instead of a burger or fries. That could mean 22–30 lost pounds a year.
- Giving up evening snacks (which you won't need because you're eating healthy meals regularly so you're not hungry in the evenings) could knock off 15 pounds.

BOTTOM LINE: Lose 20–80 pounds

This is a very significant change. I think it's clear that you can lose tremendous amounts of weight just by planning meals carefully and sticking to a regular mealtime schedule. And that's without dieting!

FACING emotions honestly and with acceptance can stop binges before they start.

■ JEALOUSY, humiliation, anger, loneliness, and boredom are uncomfortable feelings. But they're *normal* feelings. I have to stress this because the sooner you accept your feelings, whether or not you try to change them, the sooner you'll feel as though a load has been lifted from your shoulders.

No one wants to admit feeling lonely or afraid. We all want to be loved all the time, always in control of our feelings, thoroughly competent and achieving in all respects.

Sorry. Can't be done. The more we deny the ways we really feel, the more we turn to external sources of comfort, food being one of the big ones.

Larry, one of my clients, told me a story. One day in the office, he had a powerful craving for sweets. Since Larry knows himself pretty well, he guessed that the craving had more to do with his emotions than with his stomach. So he thought for a moment, and realized that the *real* reason he wanted food was because his boss had been yelling at him.

His emotions didn't change. But by understanding why he felt the way he did, his craving disappeared and he was able to avoid responding in an inappropriate way.

BOTTOM LINE: Lose 26 pounds

Larry easily saved 600 calories by not diving into the ever present plate of office cookies. Assuming he had this type of insight—and restraint—2 or 3 times a week, the year-end weight loss could be dramatic.

> **THE WAY** we talk to ourselves has a huge impact on the way we eat. Are you a perfectionist who's always self-critical? Watch out!

■ LET ME tell you about some of my clients. Julie can buy a box of chocolates and eat one tiny piece each day. Kris, on the other hand, will eat them all.

Lesson: Kris had better not keep chocolate around the house. I call this environmental control.

Here's another example. Betse asked her husband to keep the ice cream in the basement freezer so she wouldn't see it every time she opened the kitchen freezer. Another type of environmental control.

One more story. José wants to eat healthier, but he can't do it if there's nothing in the house to cook. So he plans ahead and keeps the refrigerator well stocked with delicious food that he can prepare quickly. He's learned that the only way to lose weight is to control his environment.

Everyone has different strengths, different weakness, and different food triggers. But you can see what I have in mind. Once you've identified the things that help you eat smarter, and those that send you tumbling off your diet, you can start rearranging your life to accommodate them.

BOTTOM LINE: Lose 31–46 pounds

If you do nothing more than eat healthful, home-cooked meals instead of high-fat food, you'll save at least 300 calories a night. Keep tempting sweets out of the house, and plan instead to enjoy *one* sweet *once* a week: Another 150 daily calories saved. And the list goes on and on.

A DECADE or so ago, visualization was dismissed by scientists as little more than feel-good snake oil. Well, they were wrong.

■ NO, imagining yourself thin won't solve your weight problems. But without visions of success, you are doomed. As with all things in life, you have to believe that you can be successful before you'll succeed—and one of the best ways to cement this idea in your head is to see the final results as clearly and positively as you can.

There's nothing exotic about visualization. Suppose, for example, you're hoping to lose 20 pounds. Start by visualizing yourself thin. Form a complete mental picture. Spend some time with it. Picture the outfit the slimmer you is wearing. Imagine the attention you're getting from the opposite sex. Imagine *all* the details—don't be bashful!

While you're visualizing where you'd like to be a few months or years from now, don't rush the process. The more details you create in your mind—sounds, images, textures, and so on—the more real it will seem. And that's the first step to really believing you can do it!

BOTTOM LINE: Lose 10 pounds

People who visualize weight loss—not just on occasion, but every day—will find it much easier to control temptation. Even if your positive thoughts do nothing more than give you the strength to resist a few snacks, you'll easily save 100 calories a day.

> **AMERICANS** traditionally eat a large dinner—one that we attack with zeal. Is it any wonder we gain so much weight?

■ I NEVER really understood what it meant to "attack" dinner until I watched my friend Jack. He would stop at the Chinese takeout for his favorite Hunan shrimp. He would wolf it down, all 1,000 calories, before you could say, "Let's have dinner!"

Calories that are consumed late in the day aren't burned as efficiently as those consumed earlier on. Jack's a big guy who needs about 2,500 calories daily. But he was getting almost half of them at dinner, and that was before the beer.

I asked Jack to keep a food diary for awhile. When I reviewed it, I realized that he was only getting about 300 calories at breakfast. As a result, he started getting hungry earlier and earlier in the day. He would get a full lunch, usually a burger and fries or a fried seafood platter, at an hour most people are only thinking about snacks.

This had a ripple effect. Because he was eating lunch early, there were a lot of hours to go until dinner. He found himself feeding coins into vending machines at the U.S. Capitol, where he works. But snack or no snack, he was starving by the time he left work. He'd usually grab high-calorie takeout on the way home.

A Better Balance

It was obvious that Jack needed to rearrange his day's calories, and the only way he was going to do that was to do some planning.

I advised him to start the day with 800 calories. He got it from healthy servings of granola, muslix, nuts, fruit, and milk.

We also discussed the importance of snacks to tide him over when his belly started to growl. He began to snack on fruit that he picked up at the farmers' market every Sunday, or from a street vendor on the way to work.

He was still hungry by the time lunch rolled around, but he wasn't ravenous any more. Most days, he was satisfied with a grilled chicken wrap—as long as he followed that up with some fruit in the afternoon. At night, he was able to calmly prepare himself a healthy bean and cheese burrito, or a veggie burger and soup.

Does this make sense? Everyone can enjoy a lighter dinner as long as the calories keep coming during the day. It does take some planning and probably more shopping than you may be used to, but the benefits will convince you. It works!

BOTTOM LINE: Lose 30 pounds

Eating relatively light dinners at night, and shifting more of the calories to breakfast and snacks, can easily save you 300 calories a day.

ACTUALLY, a personal pat on the back does the same thing. You've worked hard? Reward yourself, darn it!

■ AMERICANS are real demons when it comes to work and obligation, but we're not very good about rewarding ourselves for jobs well done. That's a mistake because rewards make repeat successes more likely. Psychologists call this "classical conditioning."

Let's admit, first of all, that losing weight is hard work. Cutting calories is hard. Saying no to dessert is hard. Getting out of bed on a cold morning to exercise—that's hard! Who the heck is going to keep doing all this without some rewards?

Some mornings, I find it so difficult to drag myself out of bed in order to get my workout...there's a little voice inside my head that's saying, "I'm so tired, just 30 more minutes of sleep, mmmphhh..."

But most days, I get up anyway. I do it because I know I'll feel better for the rest of the day. And to be honest, I can be pretty smug sometimes about my dedication and commitment. I give myself a mental pat on the back and say, "Good girl!" I do the same thing when I finish my workout and leave the gym. I say something like, "Thank you, God, for getting me to the gym. I feel great. (And I'm glad it's over!)"

Patting yourself on the back and giving yourself compliments may feel silly at first. But rewards are more important than you know. Instead of, "Poor me, I have to exercise," say "Exercise makes me feel great, I'm so glad I did it!" You'll be more likely to repeat the performance.

The Good-Job Club

Personal rewards are okay, but I'd rather be complimented by those around me. When you're struggling to lose weight, get some help from your friends. Insist on it, in fact.

Let's say you're getting in the habit of cooking healthful meals. Don't allow your spouse to take it for granted. Ask him (or her) to tell you how good everything tastes. (A few reminders should get the ball rolling.) Did you finish your first week at the gym? That calls for a night at the theater, or a least a bouquet of flowers.

One of my clients, Carol, is so proud of her efforts to lose weight that she asked her husband to reward her periodically—not with the traditional chocolate, but with beautiful flowers, sexy lingerie, and nights at the theater. It worked. It really kept Carol in the mood to continue losing weight and keeping fit!

BOTTOM LINE: Lose 18 pounds

Reward yourself with something that's *not* a box of chocolates once a week and you'll save at least 1,200 calories.

> **REMEMBER** the rock anthem that said "take it easy"? It's excellent advice for life in general, and it really pays off when you're trying to lose weight.

■ MAYBE it's a sign of a busy world, but we all seem to eat more quickly than we used to. You wouldn't think that plying a fast fork would contribute to weight gain, but it does.

There are sensors in the stomach that tell your brain when you've had enough to eat. But the sensors don't send "full" signals right away. There's a lag of about 20 minutes. The quicker you eat, the more likely you are to keep delivering food to the stomach long after it's had enough.

So slow down already! Rather than loading the fork as soon as it's emptied, put it down between bites. Chew each bit of food thoroughly. Give yourself time to smell it, taste it, and enjoy it.

If you do this all the time, you'll find that you're eating less than you did before. Better yet, you won't leave the table with that stuffed feeling. You'll feel satisfied, but not overwhelmed.

BOTTOM LINE: Lose 21 pounds

Eating more slowly will help you understand the difference between cravings and real hunger. Once you learn to stop eating when you're full (instead of stuffed), you can easily cut out 100 calories at lunch and dinner.

IF YOU regularly feel hungry in the afternoon and begin to forage, or if you attack your dinner as if you hadn't eaten in days, you are a candidate for a planned afternoon snack.

■ PLEASE, respond to your body's signals. If you're hungry in the afternoon, even if it's close to dinner, have something to eat. Do it now. Approaching dinner in a ravenous state is asking for a binge. (Since you've got the whole night ahead of you, it could be a real doozy!)

It is especially important to eat an afternoon snack if dinner is late. If you regularly eat dinner at 7 P.M. or later, 5 or 6 hours may pass between lunch and dinner. In that case, always plan on having an afternoon snack to take the edge off your hunger.

Amy, one of my clients, worked out in the evening, which meant that she was ferociously hungry by the time dinner rolled around. In fact, she often stopped at a fast-food restaurant on her way home from the gym—and she would consume double or triple the calories that she had managed to burn off.

Something clearly had to change. I advised Amy to eat in the late afternoon, about an hour before her workout. It might be a low-calorie frozen dinner that she brought from home and heated up in the office microwave, or the leftover sandwich she had at lunch. The snack menu didn't matter all that much, as long as it was reasonably healthy. This "mini-dinner" helped tide her over until her regular dinner at 8 or 9 P.M. Because of the snack, she was able to approach her dinner—sometimes nothing more than salad, soup, and fruit or yogurt—with relative calm.

Amy began to lose weight. The reduction in overall calories helped, but she was also successful because we customized her eating schedule.

BOTTOM LINE: Lose 30 pounds

Amy's planned snacks saved her at least 300 calories a night. She had more energy, less guilt, and more control. Way to go, snacks!

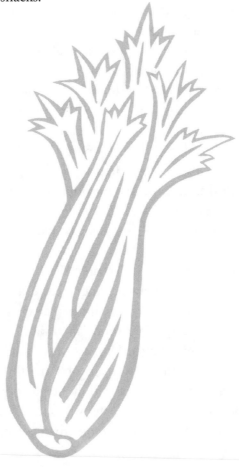

WHAT I mean is, don't go home right after work when your stress levels—and the urge to eat—are strongest. Make a little detour first.

■ ONE of my friends recently packed up and moved in order to live closer to the beach. When Linda's done with work for the day, she often stops at the beach before going home. Watching the sunset, walking along the beach or just listening to the waves gives her a chance to unwind and relax.

There must be pleasant spots in your area where you can unwind at the end of the day. Parks and river walks are great. So is (perish the thought!) dropping by the gym.

You'll notice that I'm not emphasizing the benefits of exercise. The more you give yourself a chance to unwind at the end of the day, the less likely you'll be to resort to snacking or other unhealthy habits.

Oh, don't forget to throw some casual clothes in your car. Get comfortable and have a great time!

BOTTOM LINE: Lose 15–30 pounds

A lot of my clients only take one walk a week. If you give yourself this relaxing time every day after work, the exercise alone could help you lose as much as 16 pounds in a year. And let's not forget to factor in the "anxious eating" that people often do at the end of the day. Find something else to do, and you'll save an additional 150 calories each day!

> **MILLIONS** of Americans skip breakfast, and millions of Americans are overweight. It's not a coincidence. Eating early is one of the best ways to take the edge off your hunger for the rest of the day.

■ DONNA, one of my clients, thought she had a perfect way to lose weight: skipping breakfast. The only problem: It didn't work.

When we reviewed her eating habits, the reasons became apparent. Without breakfast, she was ravenous around 10 o'clock in the morning, and would reach out to whatever was handy to satisfy her appetite. Usually that "something" was pretty darn fattening.

She's hardly alone. Studies have shown that people who skip breakfast are much more likely to gain weight than those who fill their tanks first thing in the morning.

Breakfast doesn't have to be a complicated proposition. First, have a breakfast that supplies about a third of your daily caloric needs. If you get 1,500 calories a day, then you want a breakfast with 500 calories.

Don't have much appetite in the morning? Then eat a small breakfast, and follow it up with a healthful, midmorning snack. That's what I do when I exercise right after breakfast. Most mornings, though, I don't exercise until a few hours later, so I enjoy a full breakfast. Either way, I am not hungry for lunch until 1 P.M.

BOTTOM LINE: Lose 22–30 pounds

When you eat a healthful breakfast, you'll be much less likely to load up on cheeseburgers, fries, or other high-calorie foods later on. This alone can save you 300-400 calories a day.

> **I LOVE chocolate. Candy, cookies, ice cream, you name it. But I can't have sweets every day. Neither can you, if you want to lose weight.**

■ I FIRST discovered the connection between sweets and weight during visits to my grandmother in Sweden when I was 19. She would make me hot chocolate with heavy whipping cream and cocoa. It was a perfect accompaniment to the little tray of homemade cookies she also prepared. I loved it, and I looked forward to it every evening.

Oh, and because it was midsummer, there were tender, sweet, perfectly ripe strawberries everywhere. So we sliced them up and topped them with a hefty splash of whipping cream.

I was young, which partly explains why I didn't even imagine that all of this wonderful food was going to have some unintended consequences. Foolish youth! That was when my weight problem began, and it took a long time before I figured out how to deal with it.

Sweets That Won't Be Denied

One of the best lessons I ever learned is that sweet-lovers (and we are many!) have to find ways to enjoy these lovely indulgences without negative consequences. It's not easy because sweets are high in calories relative to the feelings of fullness they provide. One luscious dessert, for example, may provide the same number of calories as a large meal with all the trimmings.

Here's what I do. When I'm going through a sweet-tooth phase, I'm going to want a treat every day. So I look for something with a reasonable number of calories—say, 120 calories per serving or less. I've found frozen chocolate bars that fit the bill perfectly. Even an ounce of good chocolate is okay.

But what if, on the other hand, I want a really luscious dessert? I plan for it and have it once a week. I'll get a lot of calories in one sitting, but that won't be a problem as long as I'm not doing it all the time.

I do draw the line in some places. A bakery near my house has some really scrumptious cookies. But once I realized that each cookie delivered about 600 calories, I decided that the long-term costs just weren't worth the pleasure. So I avoid them.

BOTTOM LINE: Lose 34 pounds

Here's some good advice. If your current dessert of choice has 500 calories, give it up, at least on a daily basis. Find a substitute that only has 120 calories. That's your "everyday" treat. What about that rich dessert? Have it once a week. You'll save 380 calories 6 days a week. That adds up to serious weight loss!

ACTUALLY, yelling is more like it. And believe me, when you crank up that cold water, you'll hear some yelling!

■ THERE ARE bath people and shower people in the world. Some of us (me, for example), are "bi"—I love to relax both ways. I spend so much time submerged in water that I hit upon an intriguing way to lose weight.

When you're finished scrubbing and are ready to exit, crank up the water to as hot a temperature as comfort allows. Luxuriate for a moment, then turn it all the way to cold. (Pause for yelling.) Stay under the cold spray for at least 10 seconds. You'll actually feel your body temperature change.

Why in the world would I suggest such torture? Very simply, it's the most relaxing treat imaginable. Unlike regular baths and showers, which leave you somewhat drained, this hot-and-cold finale will fill you with an unbelievable surge of energy.

The next time you get the urge to eat, even though you're not really hungry, you can assume that you're anxious about something. Now's the time for your bath or shower. You'll feel more relaxed and in control, and less likely to binge unnecessarily.

When I was working out my "nervous snacking" problem, some weekends I'd be in the tub five times a day! I felt it was better than nonhunger, nervous eating.

BOTTOM LINE: Lose 26–31 pounds

Use a daily shower to get you over snacking urges, and you could potentially save 250–300 calories a day.

#60 _kiss your spouse_

STRESS in personal relationships makes divorce lawyers very happy. Insult to injury, it can also make you heavier.

■ STUDIES show that happily married couples have just as much conflict as unhappy or divorced couples. The difference is that the happily married couples deal with conflicts more effectively.

I suspect they're also more likely to eat wisely, take in fewer calories, and manage their weight effectively.

I've been talking a lot about how stress, anxiety, depression, and other "negative" emotions lead us to eat more than we should, or even more than we want. Troubled relationships—not only within marriages, but also in the workplace or between friends—create tremendous amounts of stress. That's why it makes so much sense to resolve your conflicts as quickly and amicably as you can instead of escaping through food.

One of my clients, Mary, was having a terrible time at work. She just couldn't get along with her boss. Every day, she came home from work and binged.

Sound familiar? We all do this sometimes. Mary, to her credit, wanted to break the pattern. With professional guidance, she began to understand the underlying cause of her cravings, and she took active steps to resolve the conflicts. She ultimately took a new job—but even before that, she began to lose weight because she faced conflict.

BOTTOM LINE: Lose 7 pounds

Resolving conflicts instead of "solving" them with food and drink could save you 500 calories each Friday night!

IF everyone in this country would learn to relax a little more, the pounds would melt away like butter.

■ MIKE is a perfect example. A political pundit and journalist in Washington, D.C., he always faces stressful daily deadlines. One of his coping strategies is to buy a bag of candies, take it back to his desk, and devour it while working at his computer.

He wasn't eating because he was hungry. It wasn't because he had a powerful taste for this or that treat. He did it because he was tense—and if snacking allowed him to procrastinate a little, well, so much the better.

There's no question that food gives us comfort. The next time a craving comes out of nowhere, ask yourself how you're feeling. Stressed? Bored? Discouraged? All three? I guarantee you this: Start practicing stress management, and you *will* lose weight.

Back to Mike for a moment. I suggested that he practice deep diaphragmatic breathing, also called belly breathing. It's a type of breathing in which the exertion comes from the diaphragm, not the chest. It's a great stress-reduction technique because you can do it anywhere, even when you're standing in line at the checkout counter.

Mike belly breathed for a few minutes whenever he felt a craving coming on—and the craving would simply disappear. Needless to say, he started to lose weight.

Years ago, I had the habit of eating when I was anxious, and the extra weight I was carrying was evidence of how anxious I really was. Deep breathing didn't work for me. My trick was soaking in the tub. I started doing it whenever I felt the first twinge of anxiety-induced cravings. By gosh, it worked! Ever since then, I've stayed committed to this particular relaxation strategy, but also, depending on the situation, will take walks, do yoga, call a friend, flip through a magazine or talk with my significant other. My nervous eating is almost entirely a thing of the past.

Everyone has different ways of controlling stress. Communicating with a loved one is an excellent way to work out your tension. One of my clients, Elaine, always calls her sister after stressful days at work. Conversation calms her down and helps her get in control of her eating.

Another option: Consider getting a pet. Dogs, for example, are happy to take leftovers off your hands! More important, they can reduce stress just by standing near you. Research has even shown that petting a dog, cat, or another pet can lower blood pressure and help you live longer.

BOTTOM LINE: Lose 15 pounds

Once you learn to manage stress with relaxation techniques instead of by eating, you'll eat at least 150 calories less a day.

> DON'T have a dog? Then take a bath. Call your mother. Heck, clean out a kitchen drawer. Just do anything that isn't eating.

■ ONE of the most vulnerable times of day is when you first arrive home from work. You're exhausted, stressed, and hungry. Putting food in front of you at this precise time is nothing less than pure folly.

What you need to do is unwind. This might involve nothing more than changing into comfortable clothes. On really bad days, you may want to take a long bubble bath. And your dog does need to go out, right? So get moving. Blow off some of your stress. Do anything that doesn't involve the sight, smell, or taste of food. The more you relax your body and emotions, the less vulnerable you'll be to "anxious eating."

Incidentally, you might not know that people experiencing stress tend to be attracted to the fattiest foods around. You might want to plan for this by keeping plenty of healthy snack foods in the house—plenty of cut-up fresh fruit, for example, or baby carrots.

But the more you learn to unwind, the less you'll turn to food in any event. In fact, people who actively find ways to lower their stress often find that their cravings decrease at the same time.

BOTTOM LINE: Lose 22 pounds

Welcome-home relaxation techniques that divert you from chips, cheese, or other snacks could wind up saving you 300 calories—and that's every work night!

DON'T worry, I'm not suggesting something mystical. But I would like you to turn off the television, the radio, and maybe the overhead light. Get in the mood for eating.

■ MOST OF US eat on the run or while we're doing something else at the same time. This kind of automatic eating contributes a lot to weight problems.

Here's why. Your body knows when you've had enough to eat. It tells you so with "satiety signals." But we're all so busy these days, we've stopped paying attention. So we keep eating even when we don't need to eat any more.

Eliminate all distractions while eating. Stop working. Get your mind off everything but the food. If it helps, turn off the lights and light a candle. And put down that magazine, for goodness sakes!

Feeling calm? Good. Now you can focus on the food that's in front of you. Breathe in the aroma. Enjoy the taste and texture, and most of all, appreciate the peaceful space you've just created.

This process of improving awareness may feel unnatural at first, but it quickly becomes natural. You'll also find that you're much more tuned into your body's signals, including the ones that say, "You've had enough."

BOTTOM LINE: Lose 21 pounds

This type of mindful eating almost guarantees that you'll eat less than you did before. I wouldn't be surprised if you save 100 calories at every lunch and dinner.

THAT'S exactly what exercise does. It unleashes floods of chemicals in the brain that reduce anxiety and stress—and, as a bonus, help control appetite.

■ EXERCISE is an integral part of any weight-loss plan, but not only because it burns calories. Exercise makes you feel better emotionally and psychologically. And when you feel good, you're less likely to use food as a personal security blanket.

That's an important point. Unlike our ancestors, many of us hardly have to lift a finger in order to survive. We're more sedentary than ever before, and our bodies—and emotions—have paid the price. Maybe you get tired more easily than you should. Or you're always feeling stressed and under pressure. Need an emotional "fix"? Have something to eat!

One of my clients, Tom, is always ravenous after work. But he doesn't eat right away. Instead, he exercises. By the time he gets back home, his "hunger" has decreased dramatically.

How can exercise reduce hunger? Actually, it doesn't. What it does do is burn away stress and exhaustion—emotions that many of us have come to translate as "time to eat." By getting in a good workout after work, Tom found himself more relaxed and able to have a reasonable dinner instead of a pig-out.

BOTTOM LINE: Lose 30–50 pounds

Exercise can save you 300 calories of "anxiety snacking" a day. It also burns calories in its own right. Exercise daily for 30 minutes, lose at least 20 pounds a year. Exercise more, lose more weight!

IF you're having trouble losing as much weight as you want as quickly as you want, ask yourself if you've set realistic goals—or if you even care about the goals you've set.

■ NOTHING is more demoralizing than setting goals that you fail to reach. This has nothing to do with determination or discipline. You probably set the bar too high.

My advice is this. Set very modest goals at first. Even if they're so small that they seem insignificant, the satisfaction that you'll feel when you reach them will keep you going.

How do you set good goals?

Be realistic, not a perfectionist. Perfectionists can't help but fail. Permit yourself to be imperfect—and even plan imperfections in your program.

Look at behavior, not numbers. No one can "promise" to lose X amount of pounds. What you can control is your behavior. One goal, for example, might be to eat a good breakfast. Another might be to eat more vegetables. Set goals based on what you'll "do," rather than what you'll "be." Once you start doing the things that you've outlined for yourself, the weight loss will naturally fall into place.

Emphasize the positive. Instead of telling yourself what you won't do, tell yourself what you will: "I will prepare a beautiful bowl of raspberries with a dollop of whipped cream when I get home from work," or "I will go for a walk 3 days this week."

Be flexible. Exercising every day may be admirable, but unforeseen circumstances, if nothing else, will be sure to intervene. Better to make goals that are more flexible: "I will exercise 5 days every week." If it turns out that you exercise every single day, well, you get bonus points!

Set measurable goals. Specificity makes things happen. "I'll eat more vegetables" is a good goal, but how will you know you reach it? No matter what you plan to do, be specific: "I'll add a vegetable to every lunch and dinner this week," or "I'll exercise for 20 minutes" five out of seven mornings.

Make sure you care. If you consistently fail to meet certain goals, it's possible that they're the wrong ones for you. If the program you've started doesn't excite you, find one that suits you better.

BOTTOM LINE: Lose 31 pounds

Goals that are reachable will make it a lot easier to stay with the program. Even if you only reduce your calorie intake by 300 a day, you'll lose impressive amounts of weight in a year.

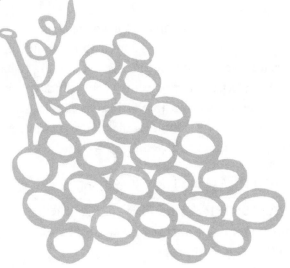

DO YOU HAVE a particular calorie-rich treat that you crave—and devour—every night? No problem. Here's how to turn cravings to your advantage.

■ ONE OF MY CLIENTS, Paul, absolutely loves sweets. He thinks about them all the time, and in the best of all possible worlds, he'd enjoy them with abandon. But none of us can do this for very long without gaining weight.

Here's what Paul does instead. Every Friday night, he allows himself to eat a rich, delicious brownie *without guilt*. In fact, he gloats about it. And no wonder. All week, from Monday through Thursday, he thinks about that brownie. Rather than surrendering to sweets during the week, he reminds himself how much he's going to enjoy that very special treat on Friday.

Is he ever tempted to stray? Of course. But he's able to resist because he knows that weight loss is all about prioritizing.

Suppose, for example, that you're going to a birthday party Saturday night. Let yourself think about the delicious cake, ice cream, and other snacks you're going to have. Then, when a sweet craving pops into your mind, remind yourself about the special treat that's still to come. It's easier to defer your desire for sweets and to make sure they're your favorites than to deny them altogether.

BOTTOM LINE: Lose 30 pounds

At 500 calories per brownie, Paul is hardly depriving himself. Yet by prioritizing his snacks, he manages to forego 2,000 weekly calories!

> **ALWAYS evaluate what works in your diet and what doesn't—and decide what you can do differently the next time.**

■ THE more you fail, the more you learn. I know, it's a tired, old bromide, but there's a lot of truth to it. People who are successful don't fail less than anyone else. They just learn from their failures, pick up the pieces, and do it better the next time.

Joanna, one of my clients, tended to emphasize the negative. "I ate too much chocolate" or "I couldn't exercise on Tuesday" was how she started most conversations.

But when I looked at her overall week, I realized that she was doing a lot of things right. Most days she ate well, exercised, and so on. When I pointed this out to her, she began to understand that she was really doing a pretty good job. Her "mistake" was that she didn't recognize her successes!

A lot of diets fail because people set goals that they don't have a prayer of achieving, like losing 30 pounds for an upcoming reunion—next month. I mean, come on! Once you realize what's realistic and what's not, you'll be in a much better position to succeed for the long haul.

BOTTOM LINE: Lose 31 pounds

People who take the time to analyze successes and failures are going to do a lot better overall. Remember, even if you only cut out 300 calories a day, you'll lose more than 30 pounds this year!

say "no" to something bad

> **PEOPLE** often find themselves gaining weight because they serve other peoples' demands at the expense of their own needs. The solution? Say no more often.

■ DO YOU work all the time? Find it difficult to turn down requests? Are you one of those people for whom the demands of career, family, or even pets always come first?

Stop! It's time to take care of yourself. De-stress and unwind. Otherwise, food will have an almost irresistible appeal. You can't eat yourself happy—but nearly everyone tries.

Here's a good exercise. Think about the things you do for others. Now, rank them. Which are the ones that irritate you the most? Now, decide which of the items you should say no to. Don't feel guilty. If you're truly irritated by something, there's a good chance that the other person should be doing it instead, without using you as a crutch.

Of course, we're all willing to help in emergencies and cases of genuine need. But that's not the issue. We're talking about dependency here.

Consider Sheila, one of my clients. She learned to say no to her boss's inappropriate demands for extra work with no extra pay. Thanks to her newfound confidence and sense of self-worth, she stopped bingeing at night—and lost 50 pounds the next year. An extreme case, certainly, but not unusual.

BOTTOM LINE: Lose 5–10 pounds

When you take care of yourself, reduce emotional frustration, and refrain from turning to food for reassurance, you'll find yourself losing weight without even trying.

IT'S often easier to say no to things that are irritating or time consuming than to say yes to things that are good for you. Isn't it time to do something nice for yourself?

■ MAYBE there's something frivolous that you've wanted to buy, or a little luxury that you think about, but are always putting off. Well, pamper yourself for a change.

True, making time for yourself may take some getting used to, but all healthy adults do it, and all say that it's worth every second. It's essential to feeling your best and living the highest quality of life possible, as well as being able to give your best to others.

What does emotional health have to do with your weight? Everything! Hunger is one reason we eat, but it's not the only one. We also eat when we're tired, discouraged, or sad. When you feel good emotionally, you're much less likely to turn to food for solace.

So what will it be? A leisurely soak in the bathtub? A long-distance call to a friend you haven't seen for awhile? Window shopping for things you like? Reading a really trashy book? I'm sure you won't have trouble thinking of something!

Oh, just be sure that your "reward" isn't food related. There are other pleasures in life, believe me.

BOTTOM LINE: Lose 5–10 pounds

Saying no to things you don't like, and yes to things you do, are the flip sides of the same emotional coin. Take care of yourself emotionally and physically. It's good for your soul as well as your weight.

6

The Party Goer's Guide to Perfect Weight

Especially appropriate for: *Party animals, Anyone who entertains (or is entertained) frequently for pleasure or business, Those who go home for the holidays*

T he social butterflies among us are very fortunate in some ways. They're often out and about, meeting new friends and entertaining old friends at home. Life is full. Life is great!

But then there's the little (or not so little) issue of weight. Festivities can put a dent in even the staunchest weight-loss resolve. Just about every party, after all, revolves around food. At the very least, there are good cheeses and other snacks, invariably accompanied by beer, wine, and other tasty libations. Just *thinking* about all the calories can make you feel heavier.

Everyone can benefit from the tips in this section, but the people I really have in mind are those who entertain (or get entertained) frequently. It's the repeat offenders who need this section most!

But let's keep things in perspective. If you socialize rarely, go ahead and splurge. Overeating on Thanksgiving Day is not going to add pounds. However, overeating on Thanksgiving *and* the following weekend certainly will. In other words, don't burn any brain cells worrying about the calories on any one special occasion. Do give some thought to your weight if your calendar is booked for days or weeks in advance.

One of my clients, Estelle, put this theory to the test. She had worked hard (successfully) to lose 30 pounds, and she had no intention of putting it back. But, like all of us, she had to learn for herself. She weighed herself after a Thanksgiving splurge. No weight gain. Emboldened by those apparently "free" calories, she splurged again, weighed herself the next day, and lo, no gain! Naturally, she went for the triple crown and splurged and weighed yet again. Uh-oh—she was up three pounds. The human body is one mysterious machine.

My feeling is that parties are a time for celebrating life and for bringing families and friends together. No one's perfect, and it seems almost antisocial to obsess over your weight when everyone around you is having such a great time. Still, parties present a lot of opportunities for overindulging. Even if you've managed to master the daily routines of exercising, eating in moderation, and so on, parties and holidays don't come around all that often. Which means we don't have as much practice reconciling social obligations with our desire to maintain the same waist size.

Okay, the social season is upon you. It is important that you take some time to plan ahead. Sometimes this means controlling your environment. Other times it means distracting yourself from the delicious edibles spread out before you.

In the following pages you'll find a lot pretty useful tips. My goal throughout is to suggest ways to have fun with your family and friends without making huge sacrifices—or gaining huge amounts of weight.

Parties are not—I repeat *not*—only about food. They should not even be *mainly* about food. Not convinced? Well, take a minute to make an inventory of the things that matter to you—that really touch your heart around special occasions and holidays. Here are some of the things that my clients have decided are important to them:

- Looking my best and feeling confident.
- The beautiful holiday decorations and music.
- Special foods that bring back memories.
- Showing kindness to others and making sacrifices for those less fortunate.
- Observing the religious significance of holidays.
- Attending holiday events, such as theater and concerts.
- Watching the kids get excited and enjoying the season to the fullest.
- Having enough free time to do special things, like going to museums or spending the morning ice skating.
- Volunteering for charitable work.

Even without knowing you personally, I can say with some confidence that your list of priorities is probably pretty similar. Do we think about food when we go to parties or celebrate the holidays? Of course. But there's also so much more.

In my experience, hosts as well as guests have a better time when social occasions aren't completely dominated by food. You won't feel bloated and heavy at the end of the evening. You won't have to worry about saying or doing something embarrassing after all of those tipsy wassails.

And, most important, you won't have to expend time, energy, or guilt thinking about how you look and feel. Now, that's worth celebrating!

> **YOU don't have to go to a bar to enjoy cheap drinks, and you certainly don't have to wake up with regrets about all the chips and beer nuts you wolfed down.**

■ WHY NOT have your next happy hour at home? It's a win-win situation. You'll have a better time with your friends when you're not getting blasted with '80s jukebox tunes. And because you'll control the food and drinks, you'll be able to keep calories to a minimum.

Happy hours are never as much fun as you think they'll be. Real conversation competes with overly loud music and the chatter of hundreds of people. There probably aren't enough stools, and you're always worrying about spilling your drink after getting bumped by the guy carrying three full pitchers of beer. Unless you're using the bar as a "meet market," it gets old pretty fast.

So have your own, after-work get-togethers. Stock up some ice and drinks. Invite friends and colleagues, and hang out for awhile. You'll all have a good time, and who knows? A little socializing with the boss just might boost your career.

You'll have to supply food, of course. Put together a feast of healthy snacks—rolled-up smoked salmon, for example, or miniature crab cakes (see recipe on page 272) and a platter of fresh fruits and vegetables.

BOTTOM LINE: Lose 33 pounds

Spend a few hours at a bar and you're almost guaranteed to consume 3,000 calories. At home, assuming you have healthy snacks and a glass of wine, count on knocking that number down to 750. Make the switch every Friday night and you'll save 2,250 calories weekly.

#71 _start a social club_

IT'S a lot of fun having a party, but it's also a lot of work. So spread the joy around. Make "home happy hours" a weekly gig, at a different house each week.

■ I'VE ALREADY talked about the impressive amount of calories you'll save by having parties at home instead of in a bar. But having a party, even a small one, can take a lot of preparation. You don't want to be the only one doing it. The solution is to get enough people involved so that no one person does all the work.

The group should be large and varied enough that it doesn't start feeling "inbred." Figure about a dozen regulars, with other friends and acquaintances showing up from time to time. Larger groups are ideal because it takes the pressure off any one person. If a few people can't make it one week, the flow won't be disrupted.

Have some friendly competition. See who can create the best tasting—or the most unusual—snacks. They have to be healthy, of course.

Even with a largish group, there will come a time when people feel that it's too much work to host a party. That's when you want to shake things up. Turn your weekly gathering into a potluck. All the host is responsible for is the wine and the venue.

BOTTOM LINE: Lose 33 pounds

Compared to the bar scene, a regular get-together with friends will probably save you about 2,250 calories—and that's just in one night. Party on!

AT the height of the holiday season, you might find yourself invited to four parties in a week. Go to all of them—and indulge at one.

■ HERE'S some rocket science: What happens when you go to four or five parties in a week, and eat yourself silly at each one? You'll make a good social impression, but the impression on the scale at the end of the week will be even more impressive.

It's difficult for serious party goers to keep calories under control. Every sideboard and dining table is loaded with food, and every bottle is filled with caloric libations.

Don't stay home, for goodness sakes. But try this little trick:

Suppose you've been invited to four gatherings. The hostess of Saturday night's party is justly renowned for her fabulous cooking. Allow yourself to indulge like crazy. Have your fill. But that's it for the week. At the other three parties, feel free to taste whatever healthful offerings happen to be available. Otherwise, limit yourself to a glass of spring water. Won't you be hungry? No, because you were wise enough to eat before leaving home.

BOTTOM LINE: Lose 9 pounds

No matter how much you eat at a special event, remind yourself that you saved at least 600 calories at the other where you practiced self-control. If you do a similar thing throughout the year, you can plan on saving a whopping 31,000 calories!

> **DON'T** waste valuable stomach space on foods you don't really care about. At every party this year, only eat the foods you really, really love.

■ THE SCENE: Platters are getting passed around the table, and you're taking a little from each one just to be polite.

The trap: You have a mound of food in front of you that an army battalion couldn't finish.

Whoa! Rein in those social impulses that push you to please others without taking care of yourself. You don't need the calories. You don't want the calories. So don't take all the food. The truth is, your fellow dinner guests could care less what's on your plate.

Next time, only serve yourself the foods you like best. It might be turkey, stuffing, and a little gravy. Or maybe you crave cranberries and pumpkin pie. Whatever. Take healthful amounts of your favorites, and pass the others, untouched, to the person on your right.

Believe me, no one's going to notice—not even the person who did the cooking. All of those staring, disapproving eyes are in your head.

BOTTOM LINE: Lose 31 pounds

Let's suppose you really pigged out on stuffing and pie. Even if you had double servings of each, that's a lot fewer calories than you'd get by sampling everything. My guess is that you'll save at least 300 calories this way. In a busy social season, that's a lot of calories!

IN order to get their fill of holiday cuisine, most people starve themselves for hours before the big event. What's wrong with this picture?

■ YOUR body needs normal amounts of food at regularly scheduled times. If you deprive your body at lunch and again at your usual suppertime, it will go into "survival" mode—and believe me, it's not pretty.

If you don't take in your usual amount of calories, the predictable result is that you're going to devour everything in sight at the first opportunity. Once the serving spoon is in your hand, you aren't going to take dainty servings. In fact, you'll easily wind up taking in more calories at one meal than you would have had you eaten your usual lunch and supper.

More bad news: Most parties occur in the late afternoon or evening. The calories you consume won't have the opportunity to be worked off. They'll be plenty busy, however. "Late" calories quickly convert to fat and make a beeline for your waistline.

Don't let this happens. Eat at your normal times before going out. Get your thrills from nonfood entertainment: good conversation, old friends, and gossip, gossip, gossip!

BOTTOM LINE: Lose 7 pounds

Keeping regular mealtimes helps ensure that you'll stay within your usual caloric parameters. If you show some restraint, you'll save at least 500 additional calories this way—and that's for just one night.

#75 *the 30-second rule*

> **THE minute you arrive at a party, pour a glass of sparkling water.**

■ "WHAT kind of wacky advice is this?" you ask. Wait, there's some science behind it.

Water takes up space in the stomach especially when it has bubbles. Studies have shown that people who drink before eating usually eat a little less, especially if they wait about 30 minutes before filling their plates.

The water serves a social function, as well. Holding the glass gives you time to relax. This is important because the urge to dive into food declines dramatically with the passage of time. You'll be more in control of your choices. You won't attack food or drink the way you would if you went to the buffet the minute you arrived, all tense from the day's frustrations.

Yes, frustrations. When people go to parties at the end of the day, they generally grab a glass of wine and a handful of cheese puffs even before they see who's in the room. "Outta my way, it's been a terrible day!"

So start out with sparkling water. Have a second glass, and then a third. Only then start looking at the food.

BOTTOM LINE: Lose 7 pounds

The typical party goer might have 2 beers (300 calories) and a plateful of snacks (another 300 calories) in the first few minutes. With my plan, you'll have water (0 calories) and probably half as many snacks (say, 150 calories). See the difference?

AS every realtor will tell you, location is everything. It works at parties, too.

■ PEOPLE congregate in the vicinity of food. They just as naturally fill their plates, whether they're hungry or not. Standing alone? A little bored? Take more food!

Hint: Don't go straight to the food table when you walk in the door. And don't stay there after you've filled your plate. The idea is to position yourself as far away from the food as you possibly can. It's a mind game, in a way: "Out of sight, out of mind" really does work. If you're not standing right next to the food, you won't be thinking about it as much, or eating it as much.

There's a convenience factor, as well. It's easy to nosh mindlessly when the food is right there at your fingertips. If you have to walk all the way across the room, you might find something better to do—maybe even talk to the person next to you!

I always tell my friends to find the most attractive member of the opposite sex and start a conversation. It doesn't have to be scintillating. Even a mild flirtation will get your mind totally off the food. And you and your friends can compare notes later!

BOTTOM LINE: Lose 4 pounds

I suspect that you can save yourself about 300 calories just by positioning yourself away from the food table. Even if you only use this trick once a week, the year-end savings will be impressive.

> **PARTICULARLY at parties, we tend to gulp food without thinking about it very much. You might be getting full—but who notices?**

■ PARTY eating tends to be unconscious eating. I want you to do the opposite and practice "mindful" eating.

Here's how it works.

Before eating anything, take the food to a table and sit down. Take three or four deep breaths and relax. Focus your full attention on the food you're eating. That goes for each bite.

If you want to talk with someone, put your food down while you talk. When you want to eat, put your full attention on the eating. Enjoy and savor every bite. Don't waste a single calorie by not paying attention to what you are eating.

Notice the point at which you feel comfortable, but not full. That's when it's time to stop eating.

I know this is hard to do in a social setting, but it works. If you're really dedicated, you'll find yourself eating less because you don't have the privacy to enjoy it as much as you know you should. That's a good place to be.

BOTTOM LINE: Lose 21 pounds

If mindful eating keeps you away from a plateful of appetizers, you can easily cut out 200 calories. Do this all the time—at home as well as at parties—and the overall calorie savings, and subsequent weight loss, will be impressive.

THE MIND is a powerful thing. Before you walk out the door, imagine in detail all the healthful things you'll do at the party. Guess what? You'll probably do them.

■ SO MANY times we succumb to situations because they "just happened." You didn't mean to eat 16 chocolate-covered pecans, but they were right there. You didn't want the extra helping of praline ice cream, but the host put it in your hand.

Hey, you're not as helpless as you think. You just didn't plan.

Before going to parties or other social events, spend some time thinking about what you want to do. Form a picture in your mind in which you're avoiding the "wrong" things: ignoring the ice cream, walking right past the buffet table, keeping your fingers out of the M&Ms bowl.

Also, imagine yourself doing the "right" things: having a fruit or vegetable snack before you leave home; grazing from the crudite platter; or simply having so much fun that food (in your mind) doesn't seem important.

Ready? Visualize success! Get a strong picture in your mind of what you want to do. You'll find that your behavior will closely follow.

BOTTOM LINE: Lose 6 pounds

My clients have told me that when they follow this technique consistently, they tend to consume about 400 calories less than they normally would. They also have a better time generally because they know they won't have to deal later on with the guilt of overeating!

#79 *give away leftovers*

> **IT'S not the holiday meal that puts the weight on. It's eating the high-fat leftovers for a week afterward. Get rid of them.**

■ I USUALLY advise people to cook big batches of food so that they'll have delicious leftovers later. But that doesn't apply to holiday meals, which are notoriously high in fat and calories. Splurging is great, but you want to get back to normal eating as soon as possible.

There are two ways to handle this. The first is to cook only enough food for the one meal. That's not easy to do because you're never sure how much people are going to eat or which dishes will be most popular.

The second option is to give away the heaviest treats. Your guests will be thrilled if you neatly wrap half a pumpkin pie and insist that they take it home. Even side dishes— the stuffing with giblet gravy, for example—will get snapped up if you offer them a new home.

You'll probably still have some leftovers—a pound or two of turkey, several sides of vegetables, and the ever present cranberry sauce. That's good. These are among the leanest dishes on the table, and you can use the leftovers to prepare nutritious, low-fat meals during the following week.

BOTTOM LINE: Lose 7 pounds

If you keep only the low calorie leftovers, they can easily replace two higher calorie meals in the coming week. That's probably a savings of 500 calories right there.

ISN'T your overall priority to look and feel your best? Keep it in mind during the holidays or when you're out and about with friends.

■ THE PEOPLE who are most successful (however you define "success") are the ones who keep their minds focused. The more you think about what really matters to you, the more likely you are to achieve your goals.

So put that party buffet out of mind for a moment. Let's focus on some of the things that you really want.

Do you like looking good? Of course you do. So do something to remind you of this priority. For example, buy a copy of *Shape* magazine or *Sports Illustrated*—the fit people may inspire you to look your best. Another trick is always to wear your best-fitting clothes: Unlike loose clothes, they'll remind you that you don't have the option of expanding.

Let's see, what else? Buy an exercise video, and keep it where you'll see it, on the nightstand or the dining room table. You might even pin up some photos of your next tropical vacation. They'll remind you of how you want to look when you're on the beach at Waikiki.

If you keep your priorities in mind during the fun times, you'll feel—and look—better all the time!

BOTTOM LINE: Lose 16 pounds

Using helpful reminders to keep your priorities front and center could easily save you 150 calories a day. Multiply that by 365, and you'll see where positive thinking will take you!

#81 *think exercise*

> **KEEPING** up your exercise routine even during the social season—especially during the holidays—will provide a great psychological edge.

■ IT'S SO EASY to excuse yourself from exercise during the party season. You just don't have time, you tell yourself. You've been good all year. Besides, it's cold outside—or not, whatever.

Excuses, excuses. We all have them, and we all tend to gain weight just when our justifications for lethargy are starting to sound believable.

Now for the hard truth. Curtailing calories is only half of the weight-loss equation. Burning calories is the other half. Give up one, and the other isn't going to be effective.

So much for the lecture. Now, let's talk about ways to get your mind back where it should be—on regular exercise. It's all a psyche game. Tell yourself, for example, "Sure, I'm going to have fun during the busy days ahead, and one reason I'm going to have so much fun is that I'm going to stick with my exercise routine. I'll have more energy, and the stress of the season won't get me down."

BOTTOM LINE: Lose 6–14 pounds

There are so many reasons to exercise: more energy, a more positive attitude, and maintaining your desired weight. Even if your exercise routine is minimal—say, walking 1 mile 3 times a week—you can count on losing 6 pounds a year. More exercise, more weight loss!

DO YOU love your friends? Then treat them as well as you'd like others to treat you—by keeping food out of sight, at least some of the time.

■ THE NEXT TIME you're hosting a party, do everyone a favor. (You're not the only one watching calories.) Rather than putting out a dozen food platters all at once, pace them. For example, bring out a big platter of shrimp. Wait until it's empty, then bring out the smoked salmon. When that's gone, bring out something else.

Everyone will eat a little less when food isn't just waiting there for the grabbing. The idea isn't for people to go hungry, but to eat at a more natural speed and rhythm and avoid mindless noshing.

This won't work for large recipes that need to be available the whole time, such as fondues or hearty stews. In this case, at least confine them to one eating area—the dining room, for example. You don't want to have food stations all over the place.

Give people, including yourself, an opportunity to get away from the constant sight and smell of food. As I've said before, food that's out of sight is out of mind. Believe me, it works!

BOTTOM LINE: Lose 7–14 pounds

Just changing the way you serve food at parties could potentially save each guest about 500–1,000 calories. Do this once a week. It's not a huge change, but even small calorie savings really add up over time.

#83 *bring out the produce*

IT'S not illegal to have fruit and vegetable party snacks between Thanksgiving and New Year's— really!

■ WE'RE accustomed to seeing baby wieners, buffalo wings, and the like at parties. That's fine. A little junk food tastes mighty good on occasion.

Just don't make it the only food. For your next party, stock up on fresh fruits and vegetables. A lot of your guests will appreciate this more than you know. People don't always admit that they're trying to eat healthier, to feel better overall, and to maintain their desired shapes and weights—but you can be sure you're not the only one who will appreciate the chance to snack on something more wholesome than a sparerib.

Because rich food is so readily available in this country, it's easy to get the idea that fruit and veggie platters are inherently less appetizing. I'd be the first to admit that a huge platter filled with carrot and celery sticks doesn't exactly set the pulse racing, but why be so limited in the first place?

Pineapple, mango, and other tropical fruits are drenched in natural sugars, and they look beautiful when sliced and layered on a plate. Cut radishes into playful shapes. Add olives for color and a hint of salt. How about a few artichokes with a low-fat dipping sauce. Delicious!

BOTTOM LINE: Lose 10–21 pounds

Put fruits and vegetables on your serving table, and eat them in place of high-fat party food. You'll save at least 100–200 calories weekly.

I REALLY don't mean that. But all too often, we think that being a good host means insisting that people refresh their glasses or take another serving of whatever.

■ YOU certainly don't want your guests going without a drink or an extra serving because they're too polite, or too shy, to ask.

But here's another point of view. Sure, they might be hesitant to take seconds, but they'll get around to it eventually. On the other hand, it's very hard for a guest to refuse a host who is foisting food or alcohol on them. The last thing they need is interference.

Go ahead and offer food or drink. Repeat the offer if you wish. After that, consider the matter closed.

I remember when one of my dinner guests refused an appetizer that I had slaved over. I was offended at first, but then I stopped and thought to myself, "Wait a minute. He's here to enjoy himself, not to please me by eating—and raving over—every bite."

Another personal story. When I was much younger, I had two dates with a man who kept pushing food on me. Once, over my objections, he even ordered extra desserts for us to share. He didn't get a third chance.

BOTTOM LINE: Lose 7–15 pounds

If you don't allow yourself to be pushed into taking more than you want, and you don't push others, you can count on cutting out 500–1,000 calories a week.

> **OVERATE? Get over it, and move on.**

■ NOBODY'S perfect. There *will* be times when you eat in ways that you'll later regret. That's no big deal—but some people are *so* self-critical! They let their discipline drop over drinks or at a party, then hate themselves the rest of the week.

I've noticed that people who are unusually hard on themselves sometimes use their failings, unconsciously, as an emotional ploy to junk the whole effort. I imagine that their internal tape goes something like this: "I was such a pig at that party last night. I never could control myself, so why bother trying? The heck with the whole thing."

If your plan crashes, and you really do want to forget the whole thing, please be honest with yourself. You may not be ready for the challenge right now. Don't hate yourself.

I think you'll realize, though, that you don't want a small mistake to derail your efforts. That would be like getting so frustrated over a flat tire that you deliberately slash the other three.

Look back at what happened. Learn from it. Use that knowledge to do better next time. Okay? Now, get on with your life.

BOTTOM LINE: Lose 21 pounds

None of my clients gets a 100 for consistency. We all goof now and then. Still, if you manage to eliminate 200 calories on most days (allowing for some slips), you'll still lose about 21 pounds in a year.

> **WE ALL need to let loose and splurge on something now and then. Do it—and use it to your advantage.**

■ SUPPOSE you have this urge for a super-duper dessert. Maybe the infamous Chocolate Cardiac Challenge at your favorite restaurant. You think about it all day. Maybe you even dream about it.

Have the dessert, by all means. But (you knew there had to be a "but") plan for it. Because the dessert is so rich, it doesn't make sense to have it in addition to your regular dinner. So have it instead. Make a real production of it. While your friends are enjoying their entrees, you can be oohing and ahhing over your succulent treat. All eyes will be on your plate, I guarantee you.

Use the same approach for all the wonderful things you enjoy. Don't give them up—substitute. Crave ice cream? Give up a second serving of sour-cream chicken. Have a taste for a chocolate shake? Don't have your usual cola in the afternoon.

Traditional diets are full of "don'ts." They take a lot of the fun out of life, and no one sticks with them very long. My feeling is you should eat what you want. If you keep your overall diet balanced and cut some calories here and there, you're going to lose weight.

BOTTOM LINE: Lose 15 pounds

If you had a full dinner plus the dessert, you'd get a whopping 1,750 calories. Give up the dinner, and your Saturday nights only cost you 750 calories. Not bad for a splurge!

> SOCIAL occasions don't have to revolve around food. You won't lose all your friends if you do something else for a change.

■ WE tend to invite friends over for dinner without really thinking about it. It's just what people do, and having a dinner party is, in some ways, the path of least resistance. It doesn't require any creativity beyond remembering what you served the last time so that you don't do it again. (That's considered as bad as wearing the same dress twice around the same people—horrors!)

Next time, get together and do something that doesn't revolve around food. If your friends aren't from the area, bone up on the history of your neighborhood and go on a walking tour. Mix it up by visiting interesting shops as well as historic spots.

Or plan a day trip together. Go to an interesting town. Visit a historic site or a music festival. Heck, rent a canoe and get some exercise! The possibilities are endless. Ideally, pick a place that's no more than 2 hours away, so you don't get car cramps.

BOTTOM LINE: Lose 6–7 pounds

You probably splurge when you're preparing a dinner for guests. By changing to a nonfood event, and eating a normal nonsplurge meal, you are probably saving 400–500 calories. Even if you only do this one night a week, you're going to see the payoff—and you'll have a lot of fun at the same time!

7
The Calorie Map for
Frequent Travelers

Especially appropriate for: *Frequent business travelers, Family or personal vacations, Visits to family or friends who keep pushing food your way, Happy-hour addicts*

Whether you're away from home on business or for pleasure, you know that traveling offers many opportunities for indulgences that can add up to extra pounds. Frequent business travelers face the greatest challenge to maintaining a proper weight, but even the once-a-year family vacation can lead to unhealthy habits that continue even when you return to your regular routine.

Everyone should be able to enjoy their travels fully while still maintaining a healthful weight. Indeed, you'll enjoy your travels even more when you know that you won't have to lose any "travel pounds" when you're back home.

I've often noticed that people tend to admire business travelers. They envy the fullness of their lives, the fact that they're constantly meeting new people, experiencing different cultures, and seeing unique sights. Travel seems exciting and exotic for those who are stuck in cubicles in boring offices.

But there's a downside. If you travel on business a lot, you know all about the harried schedules, the stress of constantly coping with new situations over which you have little control, and being wined and dined by business associates whom you don't know all that well.

Consider Jennifer, one of my clients. She travels to the far corners of the earth for her job with the World Bank. With each assignment, she never knows what conditions she'll find. She doesn't know if she will have access to a gym, or even if it's safe to walk outside. In some countries, eating fresh fruits and vegetables is not safe. She eats a lot in restaurants, which means a lot of unnecessary (and unwanted) calories. Yes, her work is fascinating, even exciting, but it also poses challenges that those of us stuck at home don't have to contend with.

Most of you probably are not frequent travelers like Jennifer, but you do have that family vacation coming up. Occasional travelers face all the same issues as business travelers. Too much restaurant food. Not enough exercise. An utter lack of fresh fruits and vegetables.

Vacations are made for indulging, of course. Nothing wrong with that. But what often happens is that the *routine* of travel continues once you get back home. You might be a little out of shape, so getting back to regular exercise is easy to put off. You've gained a few pounds that stubbornly refuse to budge. You've gotten in the habit of high-calorie eating, and getting back to a healthful routine seems like more work than it's worth.

Steve is one client who has made a concerted effort to avoid these pitfalls. Steve is an inveterate traveler. He makes it a point to trek his family of four to a different destination each year. Sometimes they travel by car. Other trips may require flying to a distant destination, where they stay put for the duration of the vacation.

Either way, Steve knows that he has to maintain the healthy practices he follows at home in order to control his weight. If he doesn't, he'll face the unhappy reality of drifting for two or three weeks in an unhealthy direction, and then fighting to shake off those bad habits once he's back home. Put another way, he can probably count on losing at least two months in his ongoing battle of the bulge. Steve wants to have fun on his vacations, to relax and enjoy them—but he's learned that an essential part of being relaxed is knowing that he's taking proper care of himself and thus avoiding a future showdown.

Even though I planned this chapter with frequent travelers in mind, the suggestions really apply to everyone. Whether you travel every month or just a few times a year, you'll find dozens of easy-to-incorporate techniques that will prevent your time on the road from taking a bite out of your diet plans.

The goal of traveling is to take a vacation from stress and boredom, *not* from the hard-won healthy practices that you've begun to employ. So with that in mind—*bon voyage!*

> **A FEW DAYS** before you travel to a new time zone, shift your meal times backward or forward, as required. You'll be less likely to slip in an "extra" meal.

■ THERE are several advantages to getting used to new time zones days before you actually board the plane. Research has shown that people who change their usual routines, including meal times, to accommodate the "new" time zone will have less jet lag and more energy.

A more important benefit, of course, is that this advance preparation keeps you from eating an extra meal on the airplane, or from eating in the middle of the night at your destination. You won't be as hungry for that second breakfast or second dinner if you're already on your new schedule.

It also helps to sleep properly before, and during, your travels. If you're on an extralong flight, you might consider taking an over-the-counter sleep aid. The idea is to shift your body clock to the new time zone as quickly as possible.

BOTTOM LINE: Lose 9 pounds

If you avoid an extra meal, either en route or after arriving at your destination, you'll save about 700 calories. You'll save even more if you manage to stick to your usual meals and snacks during the trip. Consider this: If you spend 2 days traveling and 5 days at your destination, skipping those "extra" meals could save you 4,900 calories overall. That's 1½ pounds lost (or not gained!) per week-long trip. If you travel six times a year, that's significant savings.

ENJOY the extra space and comfort. You're paying for it, after all. But try to refrain from the "bonus" foods and drinks that practically get forced on business-class customers.

■ A FIRST-CLASS or business-class transatlantic trip costs thousands. Everyone is tempted to get the most for their money—but there's no way you can stuff down $5,000 worth of food. Even if you could, do you really want the extra calories?

The food in business class is more extravagant than coach, and there's also more of it. Once it's in front of you, it's hard to resist. I recommend calling the airline in advance and requesting fresh fruit and a low-calorie entree. While you're putting in your order, let them know you only want to be offered water or diet soda, not a calorie-rich cocktail.

Also helpful: Bring along your laptop, or that novel you've been planning to read. The busier you are, the less likely you'll be to use food for entertainment.

BOTTOM LINE: Lose 7 pounds

Suppose you're flying business class from Los Angeles to New York. If you can bring yourself to give up that mini-bottle of wine or champagne, you'll save 150 calories. Forsaking the before-dinner drink will save another 150 calories; giving up one of those gourmet, "even smelling me is fattening" cookies will save at least 500 calories, and resisting the nuts will save 160 calories.

See what you get for restraint? A total savings of 960 calories—and that's just one way! Do it for each of your twelve round-trip flights and save 23,000 calories.

#90 *have a flying picnic*

EVERYONE used to complain about airline food. Now they complain about getting no food. Here's the solution to both.

■ WHY GO HUNGRY just because you're flying coach? Those little bags of snacks don't cut it. My advice: Bring along a picnic lunch or dinner. It's lower in calories. It tastes better. And it's a heck of a lot of fun.

What makes a good plane picnic? How about a deliciously seasoned chicken breast? I like cold salads—maybe some leftover white beans and shrimp. In addition to the main course, pack a ready-to-go vegetable: raw broccoli florets, for example, or, if you're feeling fancy, some chilled asparagus spears. For dessert, open a container packed with chunks of your favorite fruits. (As you've probably gathered by now, I *love* plastic containers.)

Oh, and don't forget to pack a quart bottle of your favorite spring water. In addition to quenching your thirst, you'll be able to pass up those calorie-rich beers or drinks.

BOTTOM LINE: Lose 3 pounds

Most plane picnics will total around 600 calories. That's at least 200 calories less than you'd get by eating the usual airline food, or the meals that are served in airports. Factor in the water you brought (and the alcoholic drinks you turned down), and you can count on saving 500 calories on each flight.

Put this in perspective: If you fly once a month round-trip, multiply this number by 24. That's a lot of saved calories!

WITH the added security at airports, we're all spending extra time in the terminals—usually in the vicinity of pretzel and bakery stands.

■ EATING, unfortunately, is one of the most popular ways of passing the time. The meals and snacks available at airport terminals is getting better all the time, but it's hardly getting healthier. Some might call it, um, terminal.

Consider those cinnamon buns served at most airports: 640 calories each. Those large croissants and gourmet cookies: often about 700 calories. A quick snack while you're waiting for the plane can blow your "calorie load" for the entire day.

One of the best ways to resist airport enticements is to eat before you leave home. Or at least look for food stands that offer a variety of salads or lean sandwiches. Don't go anywhere near those food carts with ready-wrapped sandwiches: They slather them with mayonnaise or other high-fat ingredients, and you have no control over what you get.

Oh, did I already mention that you don't want to get within smelling distance of those cinnamon buns? When you're hungry, the aroma will lasso you in despite your best intentions. Believe me, I know!

BOTTOM LINE: Lose 7 pounds

If you manage to circumvent the gauntlet of food carts, there's a good chance you'll save 1,000 calories each day you spend in airports. You'll do even better if you bring your own meals and snacks, rather than depending on the food served in flight. Travel once a month, multiply by 24!

#92   *steal a gym*

> **YOU RUSH to get to the airport, only to find that your flight has been delayed and you have a two-hour wait. Lucky you.**

■ YES, lucky you. The delay means that you can get in some extra exercise—assuming, that is, that you had the foresight to pack exercise clothes and shoes in your carry-on bag. I, on the other hand, travel in relaxed "exercise clothes" to make it easier.

I know, exercise isn't the first thing you have in mind when you're traveling. But it's a great way to reduce jet lag—and skim off some of those inevitable "travel calories."

If you belong to one of the airline clubs, there's a good chance they have an arrangement with a hotel gym near the airport. Or, if you're staying at a hotel near the airport and the flight delay is long enough, you can catch a shuttle back for a quick workout.

A third, slightly sneaky option is to hop a shuttle for any airport area hotel, whether or not you're staying there. I have yet to find one that actually checks that the people using the gym are registered guests. It's really no different, in principle, than using McDonalds restaurants along the interstate as "comfort stops."

BOTTOM LINE: Lose 9 pounds

Most people, left alone in the vicinity of an airport snack stand, will consume at least 1,000 calories. By exercising instead, you can count on *burning* about 270 calories. Not a bad way to use the time. Doing this once a month equals big savings.

RICH FOOD and extra meals are only part of the reason that people return from trips heavier than when they left. Exercise—or the utter lack of it—also plays a role.

■ IT'S EASY to extol the virtues of motel health clubs, but let's be honest: Most of us will never take advantage of them. That's okay because there's an even easier way to burn surplus calories between flights—by logging a mile or two in the terminal itself.

No kidding. Airport concourses are nearly as long as the runways themselves, and you'll expend about the same number of calories (9 a minute) walking as briskly as you would using a treadmill. The only challenge is to find a place to do some brisk walking without appearing as though you shoplifted a magazine and are hiding it under your coat.

Rent a baggage cart for your carry-on luggage. Load it up, then wheel the cart briskly from one end of the baggage area to the other. Or, if the weather is nice, zip back and forth on the sidewalk in front of the terminal.

BOTTOM LINE: Lose 9 pounds

Concourse exercise helps in two ways. You'll be passing up bars and snack stands, where you would have consumed a minimum of 1,000 calories. And the exercise itself will torch about 270 calories. Do this 24 times a year (figuring one round-trip excursion a month), and the weight loss will really add up.

THE RESPONSE to this advice generally goes something like this: "Why the heck would I do that? I travel to get away from home." Calm down and let me explain.

■ IT'S VERY EASY to get off schedule when you're traveling. That goes for exercise as well as meals. The problems are even more pronounced at meetings and conventions, where you have very little control over the timing of events.

What usually happens is that people get so off schedule that they become ravenous between meals. That's a bad condition to be in when you're finally confronted with decent food. No matter how much (or how little) you usually eat, see what happens when you starve yourself for a few hours, then sit down behind a full plate. It isn't pretty!

The other problem, of course, is that busy meeting schedules allow little time for exercise, and you probably forgot to bring your workout clothes in any event.

Here's a better way. If you have any flexibility at all, try not to schedule meetings at your regular meal times. Don't be shy about skipping nonessential meetings, especially those that start around 11 A.M. and continue until 2 P.M. Most conventions have tapes of sessions. Go to lunch at your usual time, and review the tape later.

If at all possible, do your exercises first thing in the morning. It's the only sure way to get them behind you. Morning is probably the only time in the day when you'll have a little bit of freedom, so take advantage of it. Besides, exercising early means that you'll have more energy throughout the day.

Ideally, you'll be in a position actually to plan the itinerary. Be kind to your fellow attendees. Discuss the need to schedule meetings that don't conflict with regular meal times, and don't start them so early that people find it difficult or impossible to get in a quick workout. Better yet, follow the lead of some leading corporations: Start off each day's schedule with a group yoga or stretching session. Attendance is optional, of course, but you'll be there to set a good example!

BOTTOM LINE: Lose 14 pounds

Sticking with a regular meal schedule will pay big dividends. You won't starve, because you'll be eating at the proper times. Plan on saving 200 calories at lunch and 200 calories at dinner. Moreover, you won't be as likely to quell your hunger pains with fatty snacks, which will save you another 190 calories. That adds up to 590 calories every day. Good job! Say you travel one week out of every month. That leaves 33,000 calories.

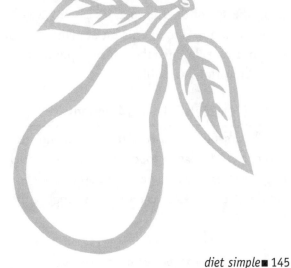

> **I'M ONLY JOKING. Most hotels are happy to arrange special meals even before guests set foot in the lobby. But you have to ask them to do it.**

■ EVEN if you're serious about losing weight, coming face-to-face with good food can send good intentions out the window. That's why I advise people to remove the threat of temptation days or weeks before they travel.

Many hotels and restaurants have begun to post their menus on the Web. Before you leave home, find out what the different hotel restaurants typically serve. What hours are they open? What's on the room service menu? Do they scale back the menu after certain hours?

Suppose you aren't thrilled with what you find. Take a few minutes to browse the Web (or, if you're into primitive technology, pick up the telephone) to see what else is available in the neighborhood. Maybe there's a seafood or vegetarian restaurant nearby, or a farmers' market downtown. Tourist bureaus are great sources of information.

In the age of the Internet, it's easy to "visit" a city before you leave home. With a little bit of planning, you can ensure that your diet doesn't take a hit simply because there aren't healthier options available.

BOTTOM LINE: Lose 14 pounds

There's no reason to settle for second best. When you consider the fat-laden food you might get stuck with, planning ahead can save you at least 200 calories at every meal. If you travel 12 weeks a year, that's a savings of 50,400 calories!

SNACKING AT HOME is easy. You probably have fresh fruit on the counter or healthy snacks in your desk drawer. When you travel, on the other hand, you won't have the same options. Or maybe you will.

■ WE'VE BEEN TALKING about the importance of planning travel meals, but it's just as important to plan travel snacks. You want to have an assortment of fruits or vegetables ready to go when you're attacked by those midafternoon hunger pangs. Otherwise, you'll have no choice but to dive into cheese-covered nachos.

When you're doing your pretrip homework, make sure that hotel room service delivers fruits and vegetables. In addition, get to know the neighborhood. Rather than checking out all the expensive fashion stores, find the delis and supermarkets. Fill a bag or two with healthful snacks, and you're ready to go for the entire week.

Oh, back to room service for a moment: If you're arriving in the evening, call ahead and make sure that a fruit or vegetable platter will be waiting in your room when you arrive. A quick snack on arrival will make it easier to eat moderately if you go out to dinner later on.

BOTTOM LINE: Lose 5 pounds

If you're on the road for a week each month, and you substitute a fruit or vegetable tray for those high-calorie snacks you might have been having, you'll easily save 200 calories a day.

> **BUSINESS** meetings are notorious for the super-caloric snacks that are offered to innocent attendees. My advice: Set a different agenda.

■ GOT extra room in your purse or briefcase? Good. It's a great place to stash healthy snacks, which you can pull out when your blood sugar drops during those interminable meetings.

During your trip, keep an eye out for fresh food at all times. If you spot a fruit bowl, grab an apple or orange. Other fresh fruit every morning at breakfast. Don't leave a restaurant without pocketing leftover raw vegetables or even breadsticks. Wrap things that need wrapping in a napkin or tinfoil, and keep them in your room. When it's time to go to a meeting, take a few of these "surprise" packages with you.

Apart from having an alternative to fatty snacks, you'll be able to keep your appetite in check all day—and you'll be much less likely to approach meals with ravenous hunger.

This is especially important in the afternoon, when so many conventions and business meetings have a "coffee break" that's also a run on the calorie bank. Have a healthful snack before entering the room. If your stomach isn't growling when the meeting begins, you'll be less tempted by those cookies and pastries that are as rich as Bill Gates.

BOTTOM LINE: Lose 5 pounds

When you substitute a fruit or vegetable snack for that high-calorie snack you might have been having, you'll easily save 200 calories a day. Do that on your week-long trips each month and it adds up!

MANY a healthful diet has gotten derailed during a multicourse banquet. Guess what? You don't have to eat everything. Nobody's going to scold you. Mom didn't cook it just for you.

■ A CLIENT of mine, Tom, once was seated next to Hillary Rodham Clinton, the former first lady and current senator, at a formal dinner. He couldn't help but notice that Mrs. Clinton didn't touch her dinner.

Tom admitted that he was a little envious. He had tried for years to manage his own weight, and leaving a full plate untouched struck him as a courageous act. But another thought also crossed his mind. Even though Mrs. Clinton totally ignored her food, no one noticed (except for Tom, who was sitting right next to her). Her restraint, he assumed, was probably a necessary defense mechanism for someone who attends multiple events on the same day.

Take a hint from Mrs. Clinton. Nobody really cares if you eat only part of your meal, or none of it, for that matter. The server gets paid for bringing a plate to you and for picking it up later. You won't get a dirty look for leaving food on your plate.

BOTTOM LINE: Lose 4–6 pounds

Consider this: If you travel frequently, there are probably a lot of occasions when you eat just to be polite. Turning down a meal that you don't really want anyway will save at least 700 calories. Do this once a month and save 8,400 calories. Do it weekly and save 36,000 calories.

YES, there really is such a thing. Who do you think arranges for all those doughnuts and pastries at office meetings? This is your chance to make a difference.

■ MODERN capitalism would collapse overnight if it weren't for committees. Nearly every decision, from choosing convention speakers to recommending "Friday fun" days at the office, comes out of committees.

So why not join (or convene) a "healthy snack" committee?

Eating healthful snacks will help you lose weight, have more energy during afternoon slumps, and generally work more efficiently. By volunteering to run this operation, you'll also avoid being assigned to tasks that will undoubtedly be dreadfully boring. Plus, your colleagues will be grateful to find some delicious, healthy choices for a change.

Believe me, you'll feel appreciated when your colleagues first catch sight of the attractively nutritious offerings. There's nothing more refreshing than a panoply of fresh pineapple served with sliced kiwi, strawberries, blueberries, pears, grapes, and bananas. Little cups of raw nuts are a good choice. So are dried fruit chips, servings of dry granola.

Bonus: Your colleagues will leave the meeting feeling great instead of miserably stuffed and in a sugar-induced coma for the rest of the day.

BOTTOM LINE: Lose 9–17 pounds

Healthful snacks make an incredible difference. Swapping a serving of fruit for the usual supercookie each week will save you at least 500 calories. Actually, you'll probably save 1,000 calories because no one stops at one cookie.

> **BUSINESS TRAVELERS** often conclude their meetings at a local bar for happy hour. You can turn these events into your greatest weight-loss opportunity—by avoiding them.

■ EVENT organizers think they're doing attendees a favor by capping days of meetings and presentations with a happy hour. It's not a terrible way to dispel pent-up emotion and tension—except, of course, for those who happen to be watching their weight. As I see it, the whole purpose of the happy hour is to blow off steam by eating and drinking—or, more accurately, by drinking and eating.

Happy hour can dump more calories into your diet than lunch and dinner combined. (Plus, many people go out to dinner *after* happy hour). An hour or two of eating and drinking can easily add up to 3,000 calories. Plus, think about all the aspirin that gets consumed the next morning. Yikes!

There's nothing wrong with enjoying happy hour on occasion, but you'll lose a lot of weight if you skip out. (You can always arrange to meet your friends at a restaurant later.) While they're at the bar scarfing beer nuts, you can be enjoying a hot shower and a TV game show or two.

BOTTOM LINE: Lose 31 pounds

Suppose you avoid 3 out-of-town happy hours a month. You'll lose about 31 pounds in a year. If you're in a hard-drinking crowd that goes out more often, you'll lose even more.

#101 *better than beer nuts*

BARS don't stay in business by selling health food. If you're lucky, you'll get a cheeseburger to accompany the beer nuts. There has to be a better way.

■ EVERYONE SNACKS when they drink—and the more you snack, the more you drink. Why do you think bars provide free, salty snacks, anyway?

Hanging out with friends at bars can be a lot of fun, but you have to find ways to reduce the calorie load. For example, put aside part of a sandwich from lunch, then eat it just before you go to the bar. Less appetite means less snacking, and less snacking means fewer calories.

Or how about drinking a tall glass of water the minute you sit down at the bar? Water will satisfy your initial thirst, which will make it easier to sip your drinks slowly, rather than pouring them down. Water also takes up room in the stomach, leaving less room for high-calorie snacks.

What if you're eating at the bar? Instead of a greasy burger, order half a pound of shrimp. Or get a vegetable plate. Traditional bars aren't likely to offer fresh fruits and vegetables, but bars attached to restaurants sometimes do.

BOTTOM LINE: Lose 31 pounds

It's easy to consume 3,000 calories at happy hours. If you drink some water, go easy on the booze, and swap the traditional bar snacks for shrimp, vegetables, or other healthful foods, you might consume about 900 calories, a savings of 2,100 calories weekly. That's worth a toast!

WANT to control your appetite at dinner? Spend half an hour in the hotel gym.

■ PEOPLE tend to eat more when they travel, and the foods they eat tend to be higher in calories than what they enjoy back home. Exercise makes all the difference.

The main advantage of exercise, of course, is that it burns calories: about 300 in 30 minutes. It's also a great stress reliever. When you're more relaxed, you'll be less likely to succumb to emotional eating and drinking.

If you exercise at the end of the day—and before slipping out to a bar—you might be content to sip a glass of water (maybe flavored with lime) or a diet soda instead of high-calorie alcoholic drinks. Your mind will be focused on health, so you'll be more likely to order a healthful snack. When dinner finally rolls around, you'll order sensibly because you already have some food in your stomach.

BOTTOM LINE: Lose 35 pounds

I've said before that happy hours are a real trap when you're trying to lose weight. But if you exercise first, and follow it up with a healthy bar snack, you might find yourself saving as much as 3,000 calories—and that's not counting the fact that you'll probably have lighter fare at dinner because you'll already have eaten something. Conservatively, that little bout of exercise might wind up saving you 2,500 calories weekly.

#103 *make faces*

I KNOW it sounds weird, but let me explain. Facial exercises will help you unwind at the end of a stressful day. That means fewer calories later on. Really.

■ EVERYONE eats more when they're stressed. Not convinced? Well, ask yourself how many times you open the refrigerator after a hard day at work. Compare it to the refrigerator raiding that occurs when you're calm. See what I mean?

Most stress-sensitive muscles are located in the head and forehead. So give them a workout. Start with your forehead. Make it wrinkle. At the same time, stretch your neck and roll your head in a circle. Now, relax.

Next, wrinkle up the muscles in your face. You can't do this exercise and look pretty. In fact, you'll look like a prune. That's good!

Next, squint your eyes. Relax them. Purse your lips. Relax them. Press your tongue to the roof of your mouth. Relax it. Hunch your shoulders. Relax them.

Now, don't you feel a lot better?

BOTTOM LINE: Lose 6 pounds

Stretching your facial muscles doesn't burn calories. But it works wonders for the emotions. By unwinding before you go to the bar or out to dinner, you'll find yourself eating in response to hunger, not tension. I've found that people who get control of their emotions often wind up consuming 400 fewer calories (that's 2 glasses of wine to "relax" and 2 slices of bread eaten nervously) during the evening than they would otherwise. Do it weekly. That adds up to a lot of pounds in a year!

HOTEL minibars are stocked by people who could care less about your weight. Those little drinks and snacks are very hard to resist. Darn, must have lost the key...

■ HUNGER strikes at all hours. Even if you're not hungry, boredom can drive you toward extra calories—and few things are more boring than being stuck in a sterile hotel room for a few hours or days. There's only one sure way to guarantee that you won't succumb to the lures of the minibar: "lose" the key.

Okay, it's a little gimmicky, but it works. "Accidentally" leave the key at the check-in desk ("Excuse me, I found this on the floor, and thought I'd better give it to you"). Don't be embarrassed—no one will suspect what you're up to!

Other options: Drop the key behind the couch cushions. Kick it under the minibar where you can't reach it. Slip it inside the pages of the *Gideon Bible*. Just get it out of sight. (But remember where you put it so you can put it back in its proper place before you check out.)

BOTTOM LINE: Lose 8 pounds

Minibars can be real killers. Even if you limit yourself to one drink and one snack, you'll tuck in an extra 300 calories. Oh, you usually have *2* drinks or *2* snacks? That's 450 calories. Spend 5 days on the road monthly, and the minibar alone will account for more than 2,200 calories.

The only solution: Lose that key!

#105 *get elastic*

> **THEY'RE** so lightweight and take up so little room that you can throw them in your luggage without throwing something else out. And they turn your hotel room into an instant gym.

■ I'M TALKING about exercise bands and tubes. Made from elastic and available in any exercise store, they take the place of dumbbells and other weights. They're all the rage today, and for good reason.

Exercise bands can be just as effective as traditional gym equipment. In fact, gyms often include them in the workout areas. The tubes can be used for arm stretches, and the bands work well for leg stretches (just follow the directions).

This type of strength training can't be beat when you're trying to lose weight. It burns a tremendous amount of calories, for starters. And as muscles get larger, they naturally burn additional calories, even when you're sitting still!

BOTTOM LINE: Lose 6 pounds

I've found that people who travel frequently often get hooked on exercise bands and tubes. The equipment makes it easy to keep up with your exercise routine no matter where you're staying. Working out in your room is quicker and more convenient than going to a gym. And we all know that regular exercise helps reduce appetite. You'll have less stress and tension. And you'll get stronger at the same time.

At a very conservative estimate, working out with elastic will save you 250 calories a day. Not bad! Do it every day of your monthly week-long trip and burn 21,000 calories in your hotel room!

I'M **NOT** suggesting that you bring that gym hunk (or doll, for you guys) with you to Cancun. The idea is to pack your favorite exercise tape in your luggage— and quit looking so disappointed!

■ SERIOUSLY, FOLKS, you don't want to disrupt your regular exercise routine while you're on the road. That's a shortcut to feeling bloated and lethargic.

My suggestion is this: Bring an audio or videotape that contains your favorite aerobics routines. Take some time every day to play the tape and get in a bit of a workout.

Hint: Call ahead to see if you can get a room with a VCR.

One of my clients, Georgia, actually lost weight on her last vacation to Mexico. Every day at noon, she put on an exercise video and had her workout on her hotel balcony in Cancun! This was a first for her—and it was the only vacation she could remember during which she actually got in better shape.

Needless to say, this is a lesson she won't forget. She plans to pack that tape, or another one like it, on all her future vacations.

BOTTOM LINE: Lose 10 pounds

Exercising regularly, no exceptions, is the only way to keep the momentum going. It's so easy to get out of the exercise habit—and once the pattern is broken, it's easy to give in to lethargic ways. The immediate benefit, of course, is that you can easily burn 400 calories a day by following the taped routines. Do it each day during your week-long monthly trip and burn 22,600 calories!

> TRAVEL, even when the final destination is exotic or restful, tends to be stressful—and stress invariably leads to eating. We could all use a personal stress-reduction manager from time to time. Well, this is your chance.

■ EXERCISE TAPES aren't the only way to curtail travel calories. Another approach is to bring along some stress-reducing yoga tapes. I can't say it often enough: Much of what passes for hunger is really nervous eating. We eat when we're bored, tired, or anxious. Control stress, control appetite. It's that simple!

Call ahead to make sure the hotel has VCRs in the rooms—or a tape player, if that's your preference. You probably already have a set time during the day when you practice yoga. During your travels, maintain the same schedule if you can. Yoga is great for centering your life and controlling out-of-control emotions. Keep it up!

Hint: Check out Om Yoga in a Box, available through the Om Yoga Center, 212-229-0267, www.omyoga.com. For $29.95, you'll get 68 flash cards, a yoga belt, tea candle, sandalwood incense and holder, and two CDs with yoga instructions and music. The flash cards have photos, stick figure diagrams, and detailed descriptions of positions. Compact for packing in your luggage.

BOTTOM LINE: Lose 7 pounds

A yoga or relaxation tape will help keep your mind and emotions centered, no matter how stressful the trip is. If listening to, or watching, a tape keeps you from having that 300-calorie snack each night during your monthly week-long trips, it has more than justified the luggage space it took up.

HOTELS usually have steam rooms and saunas. You're paying for the luxury, so use it. Relax and enjoy. You might even lose a few pounds.

■ IT'S THE END of an event-filled day in a distant city. You're tense, tired, and probably lonely. Hotels anticipate these feelings, and they surround you with "comfort"—in the form of minibars, telephones with the room-service number prominently displayed, and televisions to suck you into sedentary nights.

My advice: Confront your feelings directly. Rather than using escape mechanisms—and food, let's face it, is one of the great escapes—do everything you can to shift your feelings into a healthier mode.

When you're tense or tired, the sauna or steam room can work wonders. Take off your clothes. Get into the water or steam, and let the moist heat envelop your body. Close your eyes. You'll probably feel the tension escaping. Ommm...

Steam rooms and saunas are great any time, but they're particularly appealing on trips when you're a long way from home. The more you relax, the less you'll eat. And because saunas are located in the exercise areas of hotels, you may find yourself tempted to get in a quick workout, as well.

BOTTOM LINE: Lose 7 pounds

At the very least, steam rooms and saunas will help keep nervous eating to a minimum. Besides, the less time you spend alone in your room, the less likely you'll be to raid the minibar or order up an "extra" snack. Saves 2,100 calories each month if you travel 7 days.

> **IT'S THE END** of a busy day. Your routine is a mess, and you're lonely. What could be better than calling home?

■ I UNDERSTAND the impulse to turn to food as a way of coping with negative emotions. We all do it. Food gives us comfort. It makes us feel special and pampered. It distracts us from feelings that aren't very comfortable.

The problem, of course, is that all of this emotional eating can make us fat. If you travel a lot, you really have to be careful not to fall into this trap.

When you find yourself feeling down, discouraged or tired, don't open the minibar. Pick up the phone. Place a call to a loved one. Talk to someone you haven't talked to in months. Even a short call will make you feel better and more connected—and when you're feeling good inside, "extra" food will naturally lose some of its appeal.

BOTTOM LINE: Lose 7 pounds

It's hard to believe that picking up the telephone will help you lose weight, but trust me, it works. Look at it this way. If you feel better after a long, warm telephone call, you'll be less likely to snack for comfort. Giving up that snack can save you 300 calories a night. If you travel often, you could potentially save 25,000 calories or more in a single year. Way to go, Ma Bell!

A QUIZ: How can writing, sketching, needlepoint, or photography help you lose weight?

■ BOREDOM is among the main reasons that people gain weight when they travel. You're away from home. Time hangs heavy. You've already read *People* magazine or the same trashy novel three times. In the search for amusement, you search for food. And in America, you never have to search very long.

An easy and enjoyable way to fill the time is to bring your favorite hobby with you. By definition, hobbies are things that you enjoy doing. The hours will flash by when you're totally absorbed—and all the time that you spend engrossed with something pleasurable is time that you're not spending eating. Put another way, you'll forget all about the minibar. You'll be less likely to beg room service to empty the refrigerator and cart it up to your room. You'll stay in better shape because you won't be gaining weight.

Obviously, you won't want to bring all your equipment if you're an artist or photographer. But you can still pack the basics without consuming too much luggage space.

If you don't have a hobby, discover one. Think of activities you enjoyed as a child, even a language you'd like to learn. Research shows people who are absorbed in creative pastimes are healthier and happier.

BOTTOM LINE: Lose 7 pounds

Pursuing a hobby or favorite pastime when you're on the road almost guarantees that you'll have fewer snacks. My guess is that you can count on saving at least 300 calories a day and that's 25,000 calories a year for frequent travelers.

#111 plan your dream house

MY CLIENTS often blink when I mention this tip. "What do you mean, plan a house?" is the usual response. Wait, I'll explain.

■ "COMFORT FOOD" takes on new meanings when you're on the road. Forget it—food can be a false friend. Your goal should be to find comfort in healthier ways.

Before your next trip, jot down a "to do" list. Include some of the things that you've been wanting to do, but never got around to. Focus on fun things, like planning your dream house in the woods, writing a poem, learning to bowl, or whatever. Yes, I know there are more serious things in life, like painting the hen house. Forget it. You're supposed to be having fun, darn it!

Okay, so here you are in your hotel. Take out the list. Pick an item or two, and let your imagination run amok. Daydream, in other words.

My friend Monroe fills the time in hotels by planning his next fun vacation. He packs some guidebooks, travel literature, and maps in his luggage—all related to his next travel conquest—and he digs in. Before he knows it, he's mentally transported to Bali, or the Galapagos Islands, or Majorca. He plans his trips in great detail, and guess what? He forgets all about room service!

BOTTOM LINE: Lose 7 pounds

Creative to-do lists can keep your mind occupied for hours—hours in which you're *not* carting 300-calorie snacks back to your room or hunting down a greasy spoon just because you're bored out of your mind.

HOTEL bathrooms have all the comforts of home—except they never feel very comfortable. No wonder it's hard to relax.

■ THE NEXT TIME you're packing luggage for a vacation or business trip, make a mental note to pack bubble bath, lotion, and candles. Believe me, you'll be glad you did.

Business travel is inherently stressful, not to mention boring. It can be a challenge to fill the time in ways that don't add inches to your waist.

In a pinch, a hot shower will help you relax. But it can't begin to compare with a lazy, dreamy soak in the bathtub, especially when you've had the foresight to bring along your bubble bath, a candle or two, and maybe some fancy lotion as an after-bath luxury.

No kids storming in. No telephone calls to break the spell. Work is banished from your mind until tomorrow. You'll rarely have this sort of opportunity at home, so make the most of it on your trip.

BOTTOM LINE: Lose 4–7 pounds

If relaxing in a bubble bath keeps you from having that 300-calorie snack that you used to depend on to relax, you can count on saving at least 25,000 calories in a year.

Okay, you may feel that this special experience needs to be celebrated with a glass of champagne. You'll still save 150 calories. How many of life's pleasures can do that?

#113 *think active thoughts*

BEFORE your next trip, think about it a little differently. Visualize the active fun that you're going to have. Don't imagine huge meals.

■ DOES this sound like a parlor game? It's not. It's a psychological technique called cognitive restructuring. It means changing the way you think about things, and it can be very effective when you're trying to change your habits and lose weight.

Before your trip, don't let your mind get wrapped up in culinary anticipation. For example, don't allow yourself to visualize french fries every day on the boardwalk. Block out images of juicy steaks, or margaritas in the pool. Instead, think about active things, such as long walks on the beach or hiking a rugged trail.

The purpose of this is to get into an active frame of mind. One of my clients, Cheryl, regularly vacations in Greece. Usually she comes back with 10 extra pounds. But before the last trip, she visualized an active vacation. Guess what? She and her husband walked everywhere. They ate fresh seafood every day. It was the best vacation they'd ever had—and Cheryl brought back not a single extra pound.

BOTTOM LINE: Lose 4 pounds

Being active on vacations means you'll burn calories rather than consuming them. And you'll be eating lighter meals to support all of those activities. You will probably shave at least 500 calories a day off what you'd normally have on 4 weeks' worth of vacation. The amazing power of mind control!

FOR suburbanites especially, it's hard to imagine doing anything without hopping in the car. Well, start imagining! For your next vacation, ditch the car in favor of foot and pedal power.

■ DRIVING everywhere is an automatic reflex, but most vacation destinations offer countless possibilities for walking, pedaling, or rowing. Indeed, this is a good time to install a bike holder on your automobile—and make the bike an integral part of your vacation plans.

Before embarking on your next trip, use the Internet to scout for walking and bicycle paths, hiking trails, or canoe and kayak rental shops. Another possibility is to take walking tours, either self-guided or as part of a group. You'll be surprised at the variety of tours that you'll find—everything from ghost and architecture tours to bird-walking and history.

Most tourist Web sites will include all the information that you need. When you reach your destination, talk to motel clerks, hotel concierges, or the hosts at bed-and-breakfasts. B&B hosts are usually very knowledgeable about such things. And find the local tourist office or chamber of commerce. The information is everywhere—you just have to look for it.

BOTTOM LINE: Lose 2 pounds

Once you have an active vacation and experience the fun, you'll want to do the same kinds of things at home. The truth is that even modest increases in daily activity—walking to the store, for example—can shave 250 calories a day. On vacation, that means 2 pounds lost, instead of gained!

> VACATIONS don't have to be an "escape" from the entertainment and cultural pursuits that you enjoy at home. In fact, you'll have even more fun on the road because you'll discover what the "natives" have to offer.

■ WHAT IS IT that interests you most at home? Live theater? Movies? Art shows and exhibits? Concerts? Modern dance? The pop music scene? Ethnic neighborhood festivals? Museums? All of the above? That's what vacations are made for—explore them all!

You can do much of your preparation before you leave on your trip just by checking Web sites for your destination. Many hotels and motels have displays of tourist brochures in the lobby. You can also check with the local tourist office.

Hint: Local newspapers often have a "weekend" or "calendar" section that lists all the goings-on. Or check out the free weekly alternative papers, which are available in most metropolitan areas. These often offer the most comprehensive coverage of the local scene.

Once you narrow your list of possible activities, your only challenge will be choosing among them!

BOTTOM LINE: Lose 3 pounds

An active, fun-filled schedule is a great way to avoid "boredom" eating, so give yourself points for saving 300 calories. Plus, you'll be on the go all day, which will burn plenty of additional calories, say 400. You'll lose 3 pounds instead of gaining it!

> **WANT to make friends in new cities? Entertain yourself without spending hours in restaurants or bars? Get a heck of a workout without "exercising?" Dancing is the way to go.**

■ NO ONE thinks of dancing as exercise, but truth be told, an hour or two on the dance floor will burn more calories than a lot of traditional exercises. And it's a lot more fun.

What's your rhythm of choice? Ballroom? Vintage rock 'n' roll? Latin? Folk dancing? Cajun and zydeco? Country? Caeli? Whatever type of dancing you like to do at home, there certainly are people at your vacation destination who like it too.

David, a friend of mine, is an avid contra dancer. He always checks the Internet to learn about the dancing scene in cities on his itinerary. In fact, he tries to schedule his business trips around the dances. It's a great way to make instant friendships in a new city.

Before your trip, do some research on the Web or talk to local instructors or dance devotees. Whatever your favorite form of dance, there are probably national organizations that can steer you toward groups or even dance-based bars in different cities.

BOTTOM LINE: Lose 3–6 pounds

A night on the dance floor can burn 500–1,200 calories, depending on the type of dancing you're doing. Add in 300 calories for that evening snack that you're too busy to eat, and you can see how you'll drop a lot of weight in a hurry. Do it every night for 2 weeks, wow, what a difference!

> **THE FRESHEST, tastiest fruits and vegetables are found at local farmers' markets. While you're sightseeing, take advantage of these wonderful snacks.**

■ YOU simply cannot beat locally grown produce for taste, beauty, aroma, and nutrition. If you're traveling by car, stop at roadside stands. Stretch your legs and stock up! I really like pick-your-own farms and orchards. Long drives go a lot faster when you have a basket of berries or a bag of fruit on the seat beside you. Plus, picking the produce gives you a chance to stretch your muscles and burn a few calories at the same time.

Nearly every city has at least one farmers' market: Check the "weekend" or "calendar" section in the local newspaper. Hotel clerks and tourist officials usually know what's happening locally. Or, before your trip, check out the Internet: The U.S. Department of Agriculture posts national listings for farmers' markets. The Web address is www.ams.usda.gov/farmersmarkets. Also check out www.farmland.org, which also lists farmers' markets.

Farmers' markets offer more than just great produce. Half the fun is walking around, looking at all the people, and getting a better feel for the city you're visiting. Think of it as a walking tour, with all the fresh food you can eat!

BOTTOM LINE: Lose 3 pounds

Grocery store produce isn't always as fresh or appetizing as it could be. The produce at farmers' markets, on the other hand, is irresistible! So on your 2-week vacation, why not substitute fresh fruit or vegetable snacks for those supersize muffins, bagels, or other 500-calorie snacks.

WHEN you're on a car trip, you're almost a slave to fast-food chains and convenience stores. Fight back! Keep a well-stocked cooler in the car at all times.

■ IT'S CRAZY not to travel with a cooler. You can pack it with snacks, sandwich fixings, and plenty of cool drinks. The food you bring from home or pick up at grocery stores will be a lot more appealing than the greasy stuff that passes for food on the interstates.

Apart from ice, here are some things to consider for your cooler:

- Bottles of spring water, preferably in container sizes that will fit into your car's beverage holders.
- Sandwich fixings, such as bread, mustard, mayo, pickles, lunch meats, and so on.
- Plenty of fresh fruit and vegetables. Use plastic containers for fruit chunks or vegetable pieces.
- Greens, radishes, peppers, and other salad fixings. Don't forget a "lite" or vinaigrette dressing.
- Utensils, a can opener, plastic containers, paper plates, and seasonings.

Every time you stop at a roadside park and have a picnic, you'll be so thankful that you brought along this gear!

BOTTOM LINE: Lose 5 pounds

On a typical road trip, you might stop for fast food at lunch and at convenience stores for morning and afternoon snacks. Without even factoring in dinner, you can plan on saving 600 calories every day for 4 weeks worth of vacation.

> **HIGHWAY fatigue can be deadly. That's reason enough to take frequent breaks. And since you've stopped the car anyway, why not hike around and burn a few calories?**

■ BEFORE you leave on your trip, make sure that everyone has comfortable hiking shoes, sun protection (hats and sunscreen), and bug spray. Good, thick socks are a must.

Now that you're equipped, break up the trip with some hikes. Even the busiest interstate will have rest stops, many of which are laced with hiking trails. If you're driving on back roads, you'll find plenty of opportunities for quick hikes.

Expect some wonderful opportunities: short treks to waterfalls or scenic views, for example. In cities, you'll often find former railroad paths that have been converted to hiking and biking trails. Or make your own "trail" by following roads lined with interesting buildings.

Ideally, you'll have one hike just before lunch and another in the evening before you stop for dinner and lodging. Hiking will torch an impressive amount of calories, and the exercise will tame your food cravings at the same time. You'll also avoid "driver's lethargy"—the crash in energy that occurs when you've spent too many hours in the car.

BOTTOM LINE: Lose 15 pounds

It's amazing what a quick hike will do for your energy and your weight. A one-mile hike, for example, only takes about 15 minutes and will burn 150 calories. Do it every day of the year, including your vacations.

ALMOST everyone gains weight when they spend their vacations visiting family or friends. Politeness demands that you eat—and compliment—the food that's put in front of you. But what do you do when their food choices aren't the same as yours? The solution: Give "invisible" hints.

■ IT TOOK YEARS of visiting my grandparents and extended family in Sweden before I refined my strategy for giving polite hints about foods that I could and couldn't eat. I should have done it sooner because I always felt so uncomfortable and bloated upon my return home.

Time for the truth: These days, I usually return to the United States 2 pounds heavier than when I left. Hey, I'm not perfect! But I used to gain 5–10 pounds on those trips, and it's a lot easier to take off 2 pounds than 10.

My experience seems to be universal. When you're visiting family or close friends, they will show you how happy they are to see you by stuffing you as if you'd just escaped from a prison in Siberia. And their feelings are very, very, very fragile. "I'm on a diet" just doesn't cut it. Whether they say anything or not, what they're thinking is, "Well, if you're on a diet, Miss Goody Two-shoes, you can afford to splurge this one time. And after all the trouble I went to!"

Nothing works 100 percent of the time, but my usual approach is this: I let it "slip" that what I've really been looking forward to are those traditional foods that I never get at home. What I don't mention is that the foods just happen to be healthier than the meatballs in gravy that I usually get.

Try this on for size: "When I come to Sweden, I love to experience seafood as much as possible. It's the best in the world!" Or, before a trip to Maine: "I've been so excited because now I can eat lobster every night!" You get the idea.

Don't be shy about stating your preferences in a positive way when asked. If someone asks what you'd like for breakfast, don't feel guilty and express a preference for that fattening cheese you got before. Say something like, "Oh, in the morning I really enjoy cereal with milk, and maybe a fruit to cut up in the bowl."

It's important to keep it positive. Give your relatives the benefit of the doubt. They really do want to make you happy, even though their efforts seem misguided at times. What they want to know is *how* to make you happy. So give tons of clues and positive reinforcement ("I love your salads more than anything else!") And you'll get what you want, eventually.

BOTTOM LINE: Lose 4 pounds

If you can manage to shave 300 calories off each meal (by the standards in my family, at least, that's a very conservative estimate), you'll have a much better chance of returning home from vacation at the same weight, or nearly so, as you were when you left.

THIS is the flip side of the previous suggestion. Use positive reinforcement to let your hosts know subtly which foods you like (and which won't make you resemble a whale).

■ AS I MENTIONED before, my way of politely steering my hosts toward the foods I prefer is to innocently let slip the fact that I've been looking forward to specific (read: healthier) items.

Every now and then, they actually listen, and I make sure that they feel well rewarded. You can do the same thing. Suppose you're in the middle of a fresh salad, or a vegetable dish that isn't swimming in butter. Single out the dish for some lip-smacking compliments: "Oh, I just love salads, especially the ones with shaved carrots."

If you really want to lay it on thick, add something like, "That was delicious! We can't get anything even close to this in Washington!"

Do this consistently, and pretty soon your friends and relatives will have a fair idea of the kinds of foods you like. Notice, you never uttered turn-off words such as "healthy," "diet," or (worst of all) "low fat." By the time you're gone, your Aunt Thelma will have made a mental note that you're the niece who loves vegetables so much.

BOTTOM LINE: Lose 4 pounds

If you can convince your family to serve a few healthful dishes at every meal, you can potentially save 300 calories. Multiply that by a few meals a day, and you can see the power of stealthy hints!

#122 *stretch*

> **NO ONE** thinks of stretching as a weight-loss tool, but I know from experience that it's hard to beat.

■ HOW does stretching help you lose weight? For starters, it gives muscles that have been stuffed in car or airline seats a chance to recover—and muscles that don't hurt are muscles that don't scream at the very idea of exercise. Stretching gives a quick surge of energy, which naturally leads to thoughts of exercise. It's also a great distraction when you're starting to think about snacks.

Here's a great stretch everyone can do:
- Stand with your feet shoulder width apart.
- Keep your heels flat, your toes pointed straight ahead.
- With your knees slightly bent, bend forward at the hips. Keep your arms and neck relaxed.

Hold the stretch for 10–20 seconds. Then return to an upright position, keeping your knees slightly bent.

BOTTOM LINE: Lose 2–3 pounds

If stretching gives you the energy you need to wake up early and exercise for just 15–30 minutes, you will burn about 135–270 calories each morning. If stretching in the evening takes away your appetite for a "little" snack, you'll save 300 calories more. Lose 2–3 pounds on vacation instead of maintaining!

8
Restaurant Eating without the Bulge

Especially appropriate for: *Social butterflies, People who take frequent vacations, Business executives, Busy singles or couples, Culinary adventurers*

I love going out to restaurants. Apart from the fact that it gives me a respite from cooking (and doing dishes—ugh!), the whole ambiance is delightful. I enjoy the solicitude of the staff, watching the people, and simply taking a quiet hour or two to relax and enjoy good food.

For me, eating out is a special occasion. For millions of Americans, however, it's a way of life. I know more than a few people who eat out 5, 6, even 7 days a week. That's when restaurant food could start to present some problems.

Let's face it, one reason that the dishes we get in restaurants are so delicious is that they're swimming in richness. Chefs ladle butter on just about everything, and they choose their ingredients and cooking methods for their effects on the palate, not for their low-caloric contents. An occasional splurge won't do any lasting damage. Indulging—or, to be frank, overindulging—on a regular basis will add some serious weight if you aren't careful.

If you eat out frequently, I recommend setting some priorities. Suppose, for example, you've booked 3 dinners out this week. You certainly won't lose weight if you eat with abandon each time. What you can do, however, is decide in advance that one of those nights is going to be your "splurge night." Order anything you want. Enjoy every bite. Savor each and every one of those special calories. On the other two nights, order more carefully. Get the seafood (preferably steamed or baked) rather than the 12-ounce steak. Go easy on the cocktails. Fill up on salad rather than extra appetizers or bread. You'll still enjoy the experience of dining out, but you won't take in more calories than your diet can handle.

Obviously, you can't control what goes on in restaurant kitchens. Dishes that you think are healthy might turn out to be real calorie bombs. The only way to maintain a measure of control is to order dishes with clearly identifiable ingredients, such as sandwiches, salads, grilled meats, fish, seafood, sushi, and so on. You know that everything you order is going to be higher in fat than anything comparable that you'd make at home, but at least there won't be too many caloric surprises hiding in there.

Some diet plans forbid, or at least discourage, eating at restaurants. I can't agree. Eating out with friends is a wonderful experience. Being waited on is a joy. Professionally prepared food offers taste sensations that are hard to match. Despite all of the health benefits of homemade food, I would never advise someone to give up the pleasure of restaurants altogether.

What I do advise is eating (and ordering) smart. By all means, enjoy your meals away from home—but take a few simple steps to keep the calories under control.

Some restaurants today have websites which list calorie information. Or ask your waiter or manager if the information is available. The Center for Science in the Public Interest, a consumer group in Washington, D.C., has put together a "Restaurant Guide" which you may find helpful. Order it at their website: www.cspi.cc.

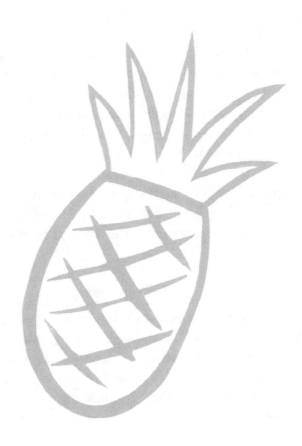

#123 *watch out for calorie creep*

LUNCH is probably the best time to eat out. Prices are lower, portions are smaller, and you have hours ahead of you in which to burn off the excess calories.

■ IF you have to choose between eating out at lunch and going out for dinner, definitely choose the lunch. You'll get fewer calories overall, and many lunch offerings—sandwiches, salads, and soups, for example—tend to be lighter than the usual dinner fare.

That said, lunch can easily turn into a caloric disaster. The main risk is from what I call "calorie creep." No matter how healthful the entree, all of the add-ons that come with it—croutons, creamy dressings, gobs of mayonnaise, french fries, or soft drinks—can change the whole equation. In fact, it's not uncommon for the calories in these little extras to exceed the calories in the main course.

Keep your orders simple. Get the sandwich, the soup, or the salad—but don't get all the extras. Drink water instead of soda. Pass on the appetizers. Ask the waiter to put the salad dressing on the side.

BOTTOM LINE: Lose 7–37 pounds

The typical burger-and-fries lunch has a whopping 1,100 calories. You'll do much better with a lean sandwich and a salad on the side—or a salad as the main course. My guess is that this will save you about 500 calories every time you eat lunch out if you make this switch. Do it once a week for a 26,000 calorie savings...or do it every work day.

THE HUMAN body is awash in water. Eliminate the water, and we'd all weigh about as much as Labrador retrievers.

■ WHICH is another way of saying that drinking water is integral to our health and well-being. It's also among the most powerful ways to control appetite and limit your daily intake of calories.

Studies have clearly shown that drinking water before a meal can dramatically reduce the amount of calories you take in. For one thing, water fills the stomach and helps send "satisfied" signals to the brain. In addition, drinking water means that you're not drinking sodas or other high-calorie beverages such as alcohol.

Speaking of alcohol, how many times have you sat down at the table and quickly downed a cocktail or a glass of wine? You may appreciate the alcohol, but undoubtedly you were also taking care of your thirst. Drinking water the minute you sit down and keeping it flowing will make it easier to drink less alcohol, or none at all.

BOTTOM LINE: Lose 4–21 pounds

A glass of wine has 100 calories. If drinking water allows you to drink two fewer glass of wine over dinner, you'll save 200 calories right there. Drink water instead of a cocktail, and you'll save 150 calories. It adds up fast!

#125 *eat simple breakfasts*

> **IF YOU** order "traditional" breakfasts at restaurants, you'll get so much fat and calories that you'll blow your diet for the entire day.

■ BACON and eggs. A sky-high stack of pancakes. Waffles drenched in butter and syrup. Is your mouth watering? Mine too! I would love to start the day with an over-the-top American breakfast, but I know too well what the consequences will be.

Of all the calories in all the meals in your day, breakfast calories are probably the easiest to control. Every restaurant, from the humblest greasy spoon to the most expensive hotel dining room, offers an abundance of healthy choices.

Hot or cold cereals, for example, are loaded with fiber. Apart from improving digestion and protecting the circulatory system, fiber is Nature's appetite suppressant. Eat a high-fiber cereal, and you'll naturally eat less later on.

Other healthful breakfast offerings include bagels, fresh fruits, and whole-grain toast. Add a glass of orange juice or skim milk, and you'll get all of the calories that you need for energy, without the excess calories that you're trying to avoid.

BOTTOM LINE: Lose 6–30 pounds

A hearty breakfast of cold cereal, 2 percent milk, fruit, and juice only provides about 500 calories—about 400 calories less than the Belgian waffle. Make this one change 5 mornings a week, and you'll lose about 30 pounds a year. Good morning!

AFTER all of this talk about the dietary dangers of meals out, I think it's worth mentioning one standard entree, seafood, that always pays off.

■ A FEW decades ago, seafood was something of a rarity on American menus. Even when fish was offered, it invariably was fried or battered beyond recognition.

Thank goodness things have changed. Today, you'll find seafood of all types—salmon, tuna, mussels, shrimp, swordfish, you name it—on just about every menu. Please, order it!

Seafood starts out so lean and low in calories that even when the dish is drenched in butter, as it probably will be, the result won't bust your buttons. You'll certainly get fewer calories than you would if you ordered a meat dish. Plus, seafood contains important fats called omega-3s, which have been shown to lower cholesterol and reduce the risk for heart disease.

If you're really being conscientious, order seafood that's grilled, broiled, or poached. It will have a lot fewer calories—and less saturated fat—than its fried counterparts.

BOTTOM LINE: Lose 22 pounds

A comparison: A 16-ounce cut of prime rib has 1,300 calories. The baked potato and sour cream that come with it add 330 calories. Oh, and the Caesar salad packs 310 calories. If you order grilled or broiled seafood and a side of vegetables instead, you'll save about 1,500 calories—and that's just in one Saturday night!

> SO MANY people have shifted toward healthier meals that restaurants have tried to make things easy by highlighting menu selections that are lower in calories.

■ TAKE advantage of them. It's an excellent way to keep an eye on your calories without having to do the math yourself.

Many restaurants work with major health organizations, such as the American Heart Association, to create meals that are much lower in fat, calories, and sodium than the usual offerings. You might see a little heart symbol on the menu, or the words "light" or "healthy."

In some cases, dishes with these symbols must meet certain dietary requirements; other times, they're more subjective. Don't abandon your common sense. A broiled chicken dish with the "light" symbol is probably a good choice, but the rules go out the window if the chef drenches it with a cheese sauce. There are no laws enforcing what the restaurant advertises.

If you're serious about watching your weight, don't be embarrassed about asking the waiter to explain what, exactly, is in a dish. It's your food. You're paying for it. You have a right to know what's in it.

BOTTOM LINE: Lose 4–10 pounds

You can assume that "light" entrees—grilled chicken with a salad, for example—will have at least 250 fewer calories than many traditional meat dishes. If you eat out frequently, making this one change could help you lose 10 pounds in a year.

UNLESS you graduated from cooking school, a lot of menu terms are probably a little mysterious. (Just what is "fricassee," anyway?) Get to know the main ones if you're serious about losing weight.

■ PEOPLE who count calories tend to spend a lot of time thinking about ingredients. They know that beef is fattier than fish. That butter packs more of a health wallop than olive oil. That chicken breast is probably a better choice than a pork chop. I can't argue with this approach, but it only tells part of the story.

Cooking techniques have just as much (or, in some cases, more) influence on the final calorie content of a dish than the ingredients themselves. Menus don't always provide clues about how dishes are prepared, but usually they do. When you see the words "fried," "sautéed," or "stir-fried," you can be sure that the dish is high in fat. "Crispy" is another danger sign.

Now, here are some "good" words: "grilled," "poached," and "steamed." What makes these cooking methods better? They require little or no added fat, which means you'll get a lot fewer calories.

BOTTOM LINE: Lose 8–40 pounds

Steamed lobster, rice pilaf, and a vegetable will have about 550 fewer calories than a *fried* seafood combo. Multiply this savings by one meal a week, and you'll lose at least 8 pounds; multiply it by 5 weekly meals, and you could lose as much as 40 pounds in a year!

> **TIME FOR A SCIENCE CLASS:** A single gram of fat contains 9 calories. Fill a tablespoon with fat, and you wind up getting about 120 calories. Oh, did I mention that salad dressings are little more than disguised fat?

■ SALADS are among the healthiest foods you can eat—but oh, the dressings! A creamy blue cheese or Thousand Island dressing almost overflows with fat. Even vinaigrettes are about two-thirds fat (the other third is vinegar).

I often get a sinking feeling when my clients describe the "healthy" salads they eat every day—drenched, in many cases, with these or other high-fat dressings. Think about the last salad you ordered in a restaurant. I'll bet that there was a little pool of dressing floating around at the bottom of the bowl. That's because restaurants normally add *way* too much dressing in order to get the desired taste.

Keep ordering salads, by all means. But ask for the dressing on the side. Dip your fork in the dressing. Take a bite of salad. Dip your fork again, and on and on. Believe me, if you do nothing else but limit the amount of dressing on your salad, you'll lose weight without even trying.

BOTTOM LINE: Lose 2–16 pounds

Let's put this dressing issue in perspective. Suppose you order a chicken Caesar salad. If you get the dressing on the side and only use about two tablespoons, you'll get at least 150 fewer calories than if you'd ordered the salad "dressed." Make the switch once a week and lose 2 pounds, everyday takes off 16.

> I ADMIT, "plenty" is a relative term. I'm not suggesting that you order a grilled steak every night. But choosing filet mignon over other, fattier cuts will save you a heck of a lot of calories.

■ THE DIET POLICE would have you believe that all beef is inherently evil, but that's simply not true. There's a remarkable variation in the amount of fat in different cuts of beef. Some cuts, it's true, contain more fat than you even want to imagine. But others are nearly as lean as chicken or pork.

The next time you eat out, pay attention to the different cuts on the menu. The ones with the most fat and calories are prime rib, New York strip, and porterhouse. Sirloin, on the other hand, is respectably lean. Filet mignon, the prize jewel at restaurants, is also lean.

This doesn't mean, of course, that every filet you see on menus is low in fat. It really depends on how the meat is served. Sauces will add tremendous amounts of calories to even the leanest cut. If you can, order your meat *sans* sauce.

BOTTOM LINE: Lose 7–70 pounds

If you order a filet mignon instead of a 12-ounce prime rib, you will save 480 calories. For those real carnivores who eat out a lot and order meat at lunch as well as dinner, those "saved" calories could help you lose 70 pounds in a year!

RESTAURANTS are well aware of the gargantuan American appetite. Most meals that you get away from home will contain enough food—and calories—for two meals. So take some home.

■ HAVE you noticed that restaurants no longer use normal-size plates? The darned things are the size of platters. Given the sheer volume of the amount of food served in restaurants today, anything smaller just doesn't work.

There's no evidence, of course, that today's humans require platter-sized portions. It's just that restaurants have gotten in the habit of serving two or three times the normal portion sizes.

Don't even try to eat it all. It's an accepted practice for diners to ask for a "doggie bag" for the leftovers. Take the extras home. Eat them for lunch the next day. Heck, you might even have enough for dinner. While you're at it, mentally thank the restaurant for its largess: You've just been served 2 (or 3) meals for the price of one!

BOTTOM LINE: Lose 6–49 pounds

Suppose that your chicken fajita has 840 calories. Eat half, and your meal will supply a respectably low 420 calories. The same principle works for that delicious shrimp in garlic sauce. Eating half and saving the rest will save you 475 calories at that one meal. Do this every time you eat out, and you'll give up a tremendous number of calories in a year.

And think of all the time you'll save by not having to cook the next day. Thanks, restaurants!

THERE isn't a law that says you have to order an entree every time you eat out. Don't take my word for it—look it up!

■ I'M BEING a little silly here, but most of the people I know are under the impression that eating out requires ordering selections from the appetizer, entree, and dessert sections of the menu.

Okay, if you're ordering from a fixed-price menu, your liberties may be abridged somewhat. But most of the time, you really do have freedom of choice. The next time you go out to eat, ask yourself this: "Am I really so hungry that I need to order every course? For that matter, do I really want the entree?"

Listen to your appetite. Maybe your hunger will be amply satisfied if you only get a dinner salad. Or soup and bread. Or even an appetizer alone, assuming the appetizers are fairly large. Don't feel coerced into ordering more than you want. You're the customer, which means that you're calling the shots. Let anarchy reign!

BOTTOM LINE: Lose 4–20 pounds

When I eat out, I might get a side order of steamed shrimp, accompanied by a salad on the side. This order will supply about 250 fewer calories than the entree with all the fixings. Even if you only eat out once a week, that could add up to 4 lost pounds a year!

#133 *have a "premeal"*

> **DO YOU** ever find yourself dreaming about a special dinner—one that's so fancy that you'd gladly starve yourself before going? Look out! Your dream is about to turn into a nightmare

■ I UNDERSTAND the temptation to eat less during the day to make room for a big meal out. It sounds reasonable, in a way. After all, if you're going to be taking in a lot of calories at night, why not cut back the calories you consume during the day?

Alas, it doesn't work. If you don't get enough calories during the day, your appetite will expand to impressive proportions. By the time you finally get to the restaurant, you'll probably order more appetizers, more drinks, and a bigger entree. Even the breadsticks won't be safe. The calories at dinner will more than offset the calories you "saved" at home.

Another problem is that you get the lion's share of your daily calories at night—and calories consumed late are more likely to be stored as fat than burned as energy. (Tossing and turning in bed doesn't count as exercise.)

My advice: Eat normally during the day. Maybe even have a snack before going out to dinner.

BOTTOM LINE: Lose 15–75 pounds

Arriving at a restaurant in a ravenous state almost guarantees you'll order an appetizer. That fried calamari packs about 1,000 calories. Eat normally during the day and skip the appetizer, and you'll automatically lose an impressive amount of weight over time.

JUST joking. You never want to annoy the person who's serving you dinner. But I do suggest shaking up the usual order of things by not ordering an entree right away.

■ THINK about all of your restaurant experiences for a moment. How many times have you been almost full by the time the entree arrived? Even if you didn't fill up on free bread and butter, the combination of appetizers and a salad may have been enough to take the edge off your appetite, or even quell it entirely.

For those who order their entrees in the usual order, there's always the doggie bag option if food is left over. But you can avoid this situation altogether by finishing the salad or soup *before* ordering the entree. You may find that by the time you're finished with the preliminary courses, you really don't need anything else. Or that a smaller entree will work just fine.

Sure, everyone else at the table will be following the script, but dare to be different. The waiter may resist, but insist. After all, there's very little extra work involved, and, after all, you're the customer. Tip appropriately.

BOTTOM LINE: Lose 6–42 pounds

Look at it this way: If starting with a salad or appetizer takes the edge off your appetite, you might wind up ordering a modest chicken dish instead of the calorically dangerous lasagna. Count on saving at least 400 calories for the evening.

#135 *start with salad*

> **I AVOID buffets. They simply offer too many opportunities for overindulging. But once you're standing in line, about all you can do is damage control.**

■ START with a salad. Carry it back to the table. Eat it slowly, and eat it all. (You did remember to get your dressing on the side, I hope!) Now, check out your appetite. You're probably still hungry, but since the salad took the edge off, you'll be able to reapproach the buffet in a rational frame of mind.

This might seem like a gimmick, but it's not. Studies have shown that when people are served (or serve themselves) more food, they eat more food. This is probably a holdover instinct from our days as cave dwellers, when food was hard to come by.

Eating the salad first gives you time to determine realistically how hungry you really are. The great thing about buffets is that you can customize your serving sizes and the variety of foods you take to accommodate your actual (not imagined) hunger.

I'm certainly not suggesting that you go hungry. But do yourself a favor and take only the food that you really need, not the amount that's required to fill 1, 2, or 3 plates.

BOTTOM LINE: Lose 3–35 pounds

The salad-first approach will easily save you 250–500 calories in a single meal. If you indulge in buffets often, you can counting on losing *at least* 15 pounds—and probably a lot more—a year!

RESEARCH has shown that when people are in groups they tend to eat more than when they're dining alone.

■ THE REASON? They're having such a good time that they're not paying attention to their natural hunger signals. And restaurants, let's face it, want you to have a good time. The more you eat and drink, the larger your bill—and the more likely you'll be to come back another time.

Eating out is supposed to be a festive occasion, of course. I would hardly suggest putting on a dour face and merely poking at the breadsticks. But you do want to focus your attention on how you feel as you eat. Are you eating because you really need the food, or are you just doing it mindlessly as part of the occasion?

Hint: Eat much more slowly than you usually do. We're often so rushed that we stuff ourselves silly long before the brain and stomach have a chance to say "enough." That's why people are more likely to feel uncomfortably full after leaving a restaurant than when they eat at home.

BOTTOM LINE: Lose 3–49 pounds

I've found that people who pay attention to their hunger signals will often quit eating when they've finished about two-thirds of their restaurant meals. This alone could save you 250–500 calories in a single meal.

9
Getting Organized and Losing Pounds

Especially appropriate for: *Hassled moms, Busy bachelors, Overworked college students, Workaholics and people who live at the office, Chefs, People who forget to eat or who eat "catch as catch can," People who don't plan their eating*

Does the phrase "catch as catch can" describe the way you eat? Maybe you have time in your life for everything *except* regular meals. You might be so busy pleasing others that your own nutritional health always takes a back seat.

I call this pattern disorganized eating. People who are disorganized eaters often feel as though they need a mother or wife to take care of them because they simply aren't able—or willing—to take care of themselves.

Well, stop it! Treat yourself as well as your mother treated you, or as well as you treat others. Aren't you worth it? A little personal mothering will go a long way toward making you feel important and nurtured. You'll notice improvements in your mood and self-confidence. You'll find yourself making healthful changes that you always wanted to make, but somehow never got around to. You'll discover how good it feels to grow as a person, to learn and to get smarter with every passing year.

I have many disorganized eaters among my clients, and they have a remarkable variety of excuses about why they find it difficult to take the time to eat properly. Take a moment and ask yourself if any of the following situations sound familiar.

- You stuff yourself every time you eat out, and you eat out a lot—not only dinner, but also breakfast and lunch— even though you never really plan to.

- You grab food whenever and wherever you see it. At the supermarket, you might be chomping away while you wait at the checkout counter. If you pass a Dunkin' Donuts, you almost feel compelled to stop. Does the expression "out of control" come to mind?

- You are so busy and focused on your work that you often forget to eat. That is, until you come face-to-face with a vending machine or join your colleagues at happy hour—and then, watch out!

- You're a college student who spends every waking hour studying or in class. You can't find the time to eat, and certainly you're never awake for breakfast. So whenever you find yourself in the vicinity of food, you grab it out of desperation.

- You are too busy taking care of your family to take care of yourself. You eat what is left over on your children's plates. You taste food while you're cooking, but you never seem to sit down for an entire meal. Still, you feel as though you're overweight and can't manage to lose a single pound.

- You're a chef or food service worker who is surrounded by food, but there's never time for a leisurely meal. The only time you can eat is at the end of the shift when all the customers are gone. You might be 30, 40, or even 50 pounds overweight. Your family is worried. Your doctor is worried. *You're* worried.

Did you find yourself in this crowd? The solution is easier than you might think. If you spend the bare minimum of time that's necessary to organize your life, you'll soon discover that you spend even less time eating than you did before. Why? Because you'll be eating healthy, and healthy eating, with a little planning, is the quickest style of eating you could ask for.

We'll talk more about finding order in chaos in just a bit. For now, I'll just say that mealtime management is 50 percent of the solution. Your willingness to try something new is the other 50 percent. Everyone I know who has taken the time to organize his or her eating swears that it saves time, saves money, and increases energy levels. Which means you'll have even *more* time to spend on the activities and people you enjoy.

A Success Story

Two of my clients, Jane and Paul, are computer professionals who spend long hours at work. When we first started talking, they were convinced that they had no time for cooking. Just about every meal was at a restaurant—except for meals that they picked up at takeout joints. After several years of living this way, Paul was 100 pounds overweight, and Jennifer tipped the scale at 50 pounds over her desired weight.

They longed for a saner existence. They knew that cooking their own meals and eating at home was an important first step—financially, if for no other reason. And when they did begin preparing meals together at home, they were delighted at the improvements they noticed in just about every part of their lives.

They started losing weight. They felt more energetic and alive. Their relationship improved because they had more quality time with each other, and that helped relieve stress and stress-related eating. They began looking forward to their evenings together, and they enjoyed planning what they might fix for dinner. The changes felt "old-fashioned," but good and very rewarding. They were mothering and nurturing each other.

The "secret" of their success was really pretty simple. Time, or the lack of it, wasn't the cause of their disorganized eating. They just needed to develop a little more focus, and also to establish some new habits. As they soon learned, eating at restaurants because of poor time management actually takes as much time, or more, than preparing meals from scratch.

An Easy Action Plan

If you're a disorganized eater, you'll need to put together a few organizational building blocks—things like scheduling regular meal times, going grocery shopping at regular intervals, stocking your office with quick (and healthful) foods, and so on.

Already feeling overwhelmed? Well, consider this. If you do nothing more than make a few of the changes that I suggest below, you're almost guaranteed to achieve the weight loss you're after. Just a few examples:

Get in the habit of batch cooking. On weekends, make large amounts of soup, stews, and main course salads. Put them in containers and store them in the refrigerator and freezer. Guess what? You've just provided yourself with delicious and nutritious alternatives to restaurant and takeout food for the coming week.

People often think that batch cooking is only useful for dinner fare. Not true. You can use similar techniques to stock up on ready-to-go lunches and breakfasts, as well.

Work exercise into your busy life. I know, no one wants to be reminded to exercise. But my clients have found some ingenious, nearly effortless ways to exercise *without* exercising. In other words, they don't necessarily belong to a gym or watch TV while pedaling a stationary bike. They incorporate physical movement—such as walking or climbing stairs—into their lives without bothering to set aside time for "formal" exercise.

Don't try to do everything at once. You'll find dozens of simple, get-organized techniques in the pages to come. Some you'll try on occasion, and some you'll use all the time. Some won't appeal to you, and others you'll love. The goal isn't to incorporate all of these strategies into your life, but only those that feel most natural for you. They're the ones you'll stick with—and the more consistent you are, the more weight you'll lose!

**DO YOU SHOP for groceries on a regular basis?
If your answer is "no," I've got some bad news.**

■ OPEN the refrigerator and take a look inside. Does yours contain only nail polish, beer, or ketchup? An empty fridge is a sure sign of shopping disarray.

Or, does your refrigerator mainly contain half-empty takeout containers, or a few bowls of moldy something-or-other? Another bad sign.

Disorganized eaters tend to be disorganized shoppers. It's that simple. When you don't have the right foods on hand and ready to go, you have no choice but to improvise. Improvised eating usually translates into splurging at restaurants or stopping at fast-food places and convenience stores. The result, of course, is weight gain.

I have two important pieces of advice. Number one, go shopping every week. Not just when the refrigerator is looking a little bare or when you've reached the bottom of the gallon of rocky road. Go every single week. It's the only way to ensure that you always have the ingredients on hand to make nutritious meals that are as quick as they are delicious.

The second piece of advice: Set a specific day and time when you'll *always* go to the store. I admit this will sound draconian to some people, but if you aren't in the habit of shopping regularly, it's the best way to get in the habit. In fact, mark the day and time on your calendar. Choose a time that works for you. Maybe early Saturday, before the hordes arrive. Later in the evening is fine, too. Whatever works best for you.

If you still aren't convinced, let me tell you about one of my clients. She was one of the most disorganized eaters ever.

Her routine—her *daily* routine—was to pick up takeout food on her way home. The meals had, on average, about 1,000 calories. I convinced her to start cooking more at home. Guess what? She saved at least 400 calories per meal. With just this one change, she lost 30 pounds in less than a year.

BOTTOM LINE: Lose 20–80 pounds

Organized shopping saves time. That's an important consideration in our busy lives. But that's just the beginning.

Good grocery shopping skills are the flip side of good meal management skills: Both save tremendous amounts of calories. Suppose, for example, you plan ahead for a daily fruit snack: By cutting back on the usual junk food, you could lose 20 pounds a year. Eat homemade lunches every day instead of stopping at the burger joint: another 22 to 30 pounds lost. Enjoy healthy dinners at home instead of splurging or doing takeout: subtract another 30 pounds.

All this just from buying groceries on schedule. Wow!

> **STRANGE ADVICE?** Well, I mean it. Life is busy, busy, busy, and if you try to do your weekday cooking on top of everything else, you'll find yourself making reservations at every joint in town.

■ TO TAKE STRESS out of your life (and calories out of your diet), you want to get in the habit of preparing batch meals ahead of time, preferably on weekends, when you're not as rushed and tired as you are during the week.

This concept is so important that I've added an extra section of recipes for batch cooking.

My clients are sometimes confused about the whole concept of batch cooking. The idea is to prepare quick-and-easy dinners ahead of time so that you always have something in the freezer or refrigerator that's ready to go on a moment's notice.

Let's say I'm going to make veal stew as my main-course "batch" meal, and broccoli salad as my "batch" side dish. I'll keep enough in the refrigerator for Sunday and Tuesday night dinners; the rest goes in the freezer for dinners on Thursday and Saturday nights.

Other nights, I might have lean burgers, burritos, or pizza—meals that I can whip up in a hurry. Since I do most of the shopping and cooking on weekends, I spend hardly any time on food preparation during the week. That makes life easy!

Let's get to specifics. For the veal stew, I want to buy enough for eight servings. I make sure that I have olive oil, herbs de Provence, and bay leaves. I'll buy four pounds of veal rump, four carrots, two onions, four ripe tomatoes, six small potatoes, and a bottle of good, dry, white wine. I don't want a cheap bottle of wine ruining my veal stew.

For my broccoli salad, I'll need a pound and a half of frozen or fresh broccoli, a box of raisins, unsalted sunflower seeds, bacon-flavored soy bits, one onion, a small container of nonfat plain yogurt, light mayo (which I already have, for my sandwiches), and small amounts of sugar and vinegar (which I already have in my cabinet).

Finally, for my quick meals, I'll need a half pound of ground lean buffalo, whole-wheat hamburger buns for the burgers (or a package of lean hot dogs and hot dog buns), a frozen pizza, and, for the burritos, whole-wheat tortillas, reduced-fat cheese, a can of black beans, and salsa.

Here's what the week's dinner schedule will look like:

SUNDAY	*Veal stew*
MONDAY	*Buffalo burgers with broccoli salad*
TUESDAY	*Veal stew*
WEDNESDAY	*Burritos with broccoli salad*
THURSDAY	*Veal stew*
FRIDAY	*Pizza and broccoli salad*
SATURDAY	*Veal stew*

BOTTOM LINE: Lose 36 pounds

Let's say you eat out one night during the week, but the other nights you have these delicious and nutritious meals at home. You'll save *at least* 400 calories per meal!

> **WHEN YOU GO** on your weekly shopping trips, you want to minimize aimless roaming down the aisles of temptation. Your goal should be to head directly for the items you plan to buy. Don't rely on memory: It will let you down every time.

■ I ADMIT IT: Index cards excite me, and I share this enthusiasm with my clients. I advise everyone to keep a few 3x5 index cards in their purses or pockets. When you think of things you need to buy, jot them down right away. I also keep a message pad in my kitchen. This way, you won't have to keep reminding yourself of things—items that you'll probably forget about by the time you get to the store.

When your shopping day rolls around, review all your notes and condense them onto one list. List food items in the order in which you'll visit those aisles or sections of the store. If you know you'll encounter the produce section first, for example, you'll want to list all the produce items together, at the beginning of your list.

This makes for a very efficient trip. You can go straight to what you want, rather than zigzagging back and forth. Apart from saving time, you'll also be less likely to indulge in "hunger shopping," which can add calories (and cost) to your weekly diet.

BOTTOM LINE: Lose 20–80 pounds

Grocery lists are absolutely essential when you're shopping on a once-a-week schedule. Take my word for it: Shopping regularly and stocking up will help you lose tremendous amounts of weight, almost without trying!

I CAN'T COUNT the number of people who tell me that they skip breakfast, and the calories that go with it, in order to lose weight. Wake up! It's a lousy idea.

■ DONNA, one of my clients, thought she had the perfect way to lose weight. She cut out breakfast altogether, except for coffee. She thought it made sense because she was eliminating all of those "extra" calories.

She didn't lose weight, of course. Whether she admitted it or not at the time, she was starving by midmorning. When she was stressed, anxious, or merely ravenous, she would grab something to satisfy her stomach. The calories from her near-constant nibbling really added up.

Donna felt guilty for her lack of discipline. But discipline had nothing to do with it. The problem was hunger and the body's demand for calories. The body has to be satisfied one way or another.

A recent study showed that most people who lose weight and keep it off successfully are breakfast eaters. That's true of adults, and it may be even more true of young people. Teenage girls who skip breakfast are more likely to be overweight or obese.

The Breakfast Habit

I understand that breakfast, for some people, isn't the most appealing meal of the day. All I can say is, too bad! If you want to lose weight, you *have* to start the day with a healthful breakfast. There are a few ways to do it.

If you wake up a little earlier than usual and give yourself enough time, you can have a full breakfast that provides a third of your daily caloric needs. If you get 1,500 calories a day, 500 of those calories should come at breakfast.

Still rushed in the morning? You might want to divide those 500 breakfast calories into two meals: Half at breakfast, and half as a healthful, midmorning snack. I do this myself when I exercise right after breakfast. Most mornings, though, I don't exercise until a few hours later, so I enjoy a full breakfast. Either way, I am not hungry for lunch until 1 P.M.

My favorite breakfast is a big bowl of oatmeal. I add milk, nuts, and fruit. I recommend this to a lot of my clients, and most find that they enjoy it. What's more, they're often amazed at how fantastic they feel after allowing themselves this old-fashioned luxury.

The bonus is, they're less hungry the entire day—even up until dinner. One of my most skeptical friends, Dan, tried the big breakfast and reluctantly agreed it controlled his appetite throught the entire day. For some people, this is the only change they need to make to lose weight and keep it off successfully.

BOTTOM LINE: Lose 22–30 pounds

If you eat a healthful breakfast every day, and the calories you take in make it possible for you to avoid "emotional snacks" or simply cheeseburgers and fries, you'll save 300–400 calories a day. Can't beat it!

BREAKFAST isn't appealing for some people. No sweat. All you have to do is create an office breakfast stash. It's ready whenever you are!

■ PERHAPS you just don't feel like eating when you first get up. My friend Linda is like that—but she doesn't let it stop her from having a nutritious, filling breakfast.

"I'm not a morning person and I could never get interested in eating breakfast until I started bringing it to work," she says. "On Mondays, I bring in a loaf of my favorite grain bread, a large container of cottage cheese, a box of instant oatmeal, and some fresh fruit that lasts, like apples and pears. I leave everything at the office for the week. With a fridge and microwave at the office, it's no sweat for me to make a nice breakfast when I'm finally hungry, usually around 9 A.M."

Almost everything you normally eat at home can also be enjoyed at the office. Most offices have microwaves, so you can even have some turkey bacon or a veggie sausage. How about whole grain toast with peanut butter and a serving of fresh fruit? Or cereal with milk and fresh fruit?

Even if you don't have access to a refrigerator, there are plenty of wholesome breakfast foods that will fit in a desk drawer, such as minicontainers of cereal, raisins, or high-fiber crackers.

BOTTOM LINE: Lose 22–30 pounds

A satisfying office breakfast can stave off cravings for a cheeseburger and fries—and save you 300–400 calories every day.

#142 *cook more than you can eat*

A STRANGE suggestion to find in a weight-loss book? Believe it or not, it's among the best approaches for shedding extra pounds because the foods you cook today become nutritious leftovers for later.

■ IN OUR FRENZIED super-busy world, time is the most precious commodity. We never have enough of it. That's why it is so tempting to cut corners and pick up something to eat at a drive-up window on the way home.

My advice: Make the most of the time you spend in the kitchen. Make more than you can eat now. Put what's left in the refrigerator or freezer. You'll be surprised how just knowing that something delicious is waiting for you staves off temptation on the way home. It also makes it possible to invite a friend over at the last moment rather than going out together to eat.

Having food that's ready to go is one of the most important steps you can take, and it's one of the most important tips in this book. It can save you hundreds of calories each and every night because you'll be less likely to order high-fat meals at restaurants. That can add up to plenty of lost pounds in a year's time, or even a month's time.

BOTTOM LINE: Lose 30–42 pounds

A meal at a restaurant or fast-food joint will easily set you back 1,000 calories. A meal cooked at home, including those delicious leftovers, has only about 600 calories. So cook more—and cook large!

> **FRESH** fruits and vegetables are deliciously whole-some, but frozen or ready-cut produce are every bit as good—and they're more convenient.

■ YOU ALREADY KNOW how nutritious fruits and vegetables are, so I don't have to sell you on that. The most important thing is to eat a variety of fruits and vegetables, preferably with every meal.

Don't fret about always getting your fruits and vegetables fresh. In the summer, I buy as much as I can from the farmers' market. In the winter, I get all my produce at the grocery store—fresh, frozen, or canned. The advantage of frozen and canned fruits and vegetables is that they're usually picked when perfectly ripe, then frozen or canned immediately. "Fresh" grocery store produce, on the other hand, is often picked early to compensate for the long storage times. Frozen is often the most convenient choice because it's been cleaned and chopped into bite sizes.

When buying fresh: Consider cleaning, chopping, and storing fresh produce in plastic containers or baggies as soon as you get home. That way, it's ready for use all week long. As long as you eat it every day, you won't run the risk of turning your refrigerator crisper into a "rotter." And your kids will have healthy snacks they can grab any time.

BOTTOM LINE: Lose up to 20–50 pounds

If you add a salad to your evening meal, and cut back on portion sizes generally, you can lose 30 pounds in a year. Substituting a fruit snack for a vending machine snack every day will save another 20 pounds!

#144 *eat more to eat less*

THE BIGGEST cause of overeating is undereating. No kidding. People often go too long without eating, then pig out when they're ravenously hungry. Call it poor mealtime management.

■ YOUR BODY is designed to get hungry every 3 to 4 hours. The traditional, 3-meal-a-day plan is about the worst way to eat. It is much better to have a regular progression of meals: breakfast, snack, lunch, snack, and dinner.

This sort of regular routine maintains your body's normal hunger signals. It also boosts the metabolism to its highest rates, making it more efficient at burning calories.

Unfortunately, we tend to focus most of our attention on a few big meals, especially dinner. That's a problem because your body needs calories during the day, when you're active and burning them. It doesn't need large amounts of calories at night, when the body's natural rhythm is to slow down.

Research shows that people who eat their largest meal at night tend to be more overweight and have higher cholesterol levels than those who eat smaller amounts of food throughout the day.

Also, eating more often—and including planned snacks in your routine—is a great way to prevent binges. Binges usually are a result of poor planning: You'll inevitably find yourself at a wrong place (a fast-food restaurant, a vending machine) at the wrong time (when you're ravenous).

A Better Way

Here's what I advise nearly all of my clients:

- Eat your usual supper at least three hours before going to bed. Make this your last meal of the day, if you can.
- Allow for exceptions. You want to eat when you're hungry, and if for some reason you're truly hungry after supper— and you're not merely bored, tired, or depressed—go ahead and have a snack. A piece of fresh fruit is best. Or vegetables, which make a great snack at any time.
- Always plan to have a snack in midmorning and midafternoon. Your body needs the calories—listen to it!

If you do nothing else except plan your meals more carefully, *you're going to lose weight*. I guarantee it. In fact, the amount of weight you'll lose over a year, even if this is all you do, will be impressive.

BOTTOM LINE: Lose 20–50 pounds

The great thing about mealtime management is that it doesn't involve dieting. All you're doing is eating delicious food at the right times! Some examples: Regular meals can eliminate the need for high-calorie snacks; planning for a fruit snack instead of raiding the doughnut box can melt away 20 pounds; and planning a healthful lunch instead of grabbing something on the fly can help you lose 22–30 pounds a year.

YOU'VE BEEN GOOD about substituting lean roast beef or chicken sandwiches for hamburgers, but your cravings can no longer be denied. Don't feel guilty—enjoy!

■ HAMBURGERS have gotten a bad rap. As long as you make them at home (rather than *bringing* them home), they're low enough in fat to eat all the time. You can even add Thousand Island dressing for a faux Big Mac.

Put this in perspective: A half pound of burger meat at your favorite burger joint will set you back 800 calories. If you buy extra-lean ground meat and make your own, you'll get 200 calories less.

Better yet: Buy a round steak, have the butcher remove the visible fat, and ask him to grind the rest. This meat is 95 percent lean or better—the equivalent of game meat like venison or buffalo. You're down to 400 calories, half the amount in the takeout.

The calories in lettuce, tomato, pickles, and so on hardly register. As for dressing, I prefer the regular mayonnaise. Even though it has 100 calories (compared to the 50 in low-fat), the meat-substitute trick keeps the whole thing in the safety zone.

To make your burger healthier, use whole-grain bread or buns instead of that nutritional disaster known as white bread.

BOTTOM LINE: Lose 6–18 pounds

Making your own burgers weekly with lean meat and healthy fixings means that you can enjoy them all the time—with only a fraction of the calories that you'd get in ready-made. Make the switch often and lose even more.

> **MOST OF US** spend more time at the office than at home. The ready availability of fast food, vending machine snacks, and morning doughnuts offer bounteous opportunities for expanding our waistlines.

■ THE TYPICAL WORKDAY and workplace are almost perfectly designed for gaining weight. Morning is too rushed to eat a proper breakfast, so we stop at a convenience store or fast-food restaurant for a quick (and high-fat) meal. We go out to lunch with colleagues, or ask one of them to bring back a burger meal to eat at our desks. We drop quarters in vending machines for afternoon snacks. And on those days when we work late (and we all have them), we can't face the thought of preparing dinner at home, so we end up, again, at a restaurant or fast-food chain.

Here's a better way.

Most offices today have communal kitchens, with a refrigerator, stove, and microwave. Take advantage of this corporate largess by bringing your own supplies—not only quick snacks, such as pretzels and dried fruit, but also complete meals, which you can prepare whenever you're in the mood for something healthier than the usual office or takeout fare.

It's easier than it sounds. By preparing meals ahead of time and storing them in plastic bags or containers in your office refrigerator, you'll always have delicious and nutritious meals and snacks at your fingertips.

Unfortunately, every office has its share of hungry predators—you know, the ones who won't think twice about raiding your healthful stash.

Hint: Try putting a "poison" sign on your food containers. And if *that* doesn't keep the rats out, buy a small refrigerator or cabinet and keep it in your office space.

Let's take a look at some of the payoffs:

- You'll save a lot of time when you don't go out to eat.
- Buying groceries is less expensive than eating out. You're paying dearly for that "convenience," you know.
- You'll almost automatically lose weight because you won't be eating calorie-rich burgers or takeout food.

BOTTOM LINE: Lose 11–60 pounds

At the office you can expect to save at least 300 calories when you prepare your own lunch; 150 calories by bringing your own afternoon snack; and more than 400 calories by eating your own delicious dinner instead of grabbing chow at a takeout dive. Dramatic savings—and that's without going on a diet!

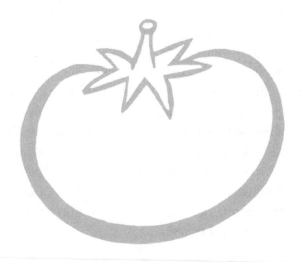

FOR A LONG TIME, plastic was a dirty word. Today we know how to use plastic to help us eat less.

■ PORTION CONTROL is one of the biggest challenges when you're trying to lose weight. When you use plastic containers, portion control is almost guaranteed: What doesn't fit inside a single-serving container is saved for another day!

Another benefit: You can put leftovers in plastic storage containers and take them to work—or keep them in the refrigerator for those busy days when you're on the go. It's a great way to avoid becoming a "vending machine victim." In the long run, the wise use of plastic containers will help you eat less, lose weight, and potentially save hundreds of dollars a month.

Also, this is an exciting time for plastics. New products make it possible to write the date and contents directly on the container. You'll always know what's inside, and how fresh (or ancient!) it is.

My personal favorite use of plastic is the "salad shaker." You keep the veggies in the larger compartment on the bottom, and put the dressing (vinaigrette, of course) in the compartment above. When you're ready to eat, simply release the dressing and shake. No more soggy salad!

BOTTOM LINE: Lose 10–40 pounds

When you use plastic containers to store meals—especially batch meals that you prepare ahead of time—you'll give up all those calories that come from greasy spoon diners. Go, plastics!

#148 *shop online*

ALL GROCERIES aren't created equal. Doing your shopping online can save impressive amounts of time—and calories.

■ IF YOU aren't entirely comfortable with the world of the Internet, the idea of buying fruits, vegetables, meats, or seafood online may seem pretty strange. No matter how enticing and colorful the pictures on your monitor are, they aren't the same tomatoes or steaks that you're actually putting in your grocery bag! No question, grocery shopping on your computer isn't the same as pushing the cart yourself.

But please, consider it. It's a very attractive option, especially when you're trying to stay organized. There's no substitute for shopping regularly and keeping the larder well stocked when you're trying to lose weight.

Shopping online is a great way to save valuable time—and, as we've seen, convenience and time savings are at the core of organized, healthful eating. It's true that online grocery deliveries require you to be home at a specified time, but you may be able to schedule the delivery for a time you're going to be home anyway.

Think about it: If you don't physically go to the supermarket, you have more time to enjoy dinner with your family. True, you'll pay for this convenience with a delivery fee—but the fee is almost certainly less than what you pay a babysitter when you take off to run errands.

What to look for:

■ Does the online grocer have the exact products you want, in the sizes and formulations you prefer? These companies have thousands of items, but not as many variations as the supermarket down the street.

- How good and prompt is the delivery service? Is the delivery charge reasonable?
- Do they get your order right? For example, are the steaks and produce equal in quality to those you'd pick out yourself?
- Does the company offer the same specials and bonuses as the supermarket you usually go to?
- Is the Web site easy to navigate? More important, are the time savings worth the loss of control over the shopping experience?

Carole Sugarman, a writer for the *Washington Post*, compared two online grocers, HomeRuns.com and Peapod.com. She liked both. You will want to do some comparison shopping at the beginning, too.

BOTTOM LINE: Lose 20–80 pounds

Your main considerations will probably be convenience and time savings. The weight-loss benefit should be the same as with physically going to the grocery store once a week. Not bad!

#149 *slash corporate calories*

SAD BUT TRUE: Too many of us work late at the office—and fast-food joints have reaped the windfall.

■ IF YOU often stay late at work, it's a good idea to have a few dinner items stored in the office freezer. A frozen dinner or made-at-home batch meal will be piping hot in minutes. You'll get your work done without sacrificing good nutrition or the comfort of a good meal at the end of the day.

Of course, if you prepared a hot lunch, you can use some of the same ingredients to make a delicious cold sandwich for dinner. There's no law that says you have to have your big, hot meal at night. Actually, the opposite is better for you: When you have your main meal at lunch, your body has more active hours to burn off the calories.

My friend Catherine brings frozen dinner meals and vegetables to work at the beginning of the week. She often gets frozen vegetables prepared in a butter sauce: She likes the taste—and because she saves so many calories by not going to restaurants, she can afford the extra indulgence.

BOTTOM LINE: Lose 6–18 pounds

Office-prepared dinners will easily have 400 fewer calories than restaurant meals. If you work late an average of 3 times a week, this change alone will help you lose about 18 pounds. Those who work late every night could potentially lose 30 pounds a year—but I'd probably advise them to look for a new job!

> **FORGET DOUGHNUTS** and other office snacks: An all-American lunch will save loads of calories, satisfy your appetite, and keep your energy high.

■ WHAT'S an all-American lunch? Well, you probably can imagine 50 variations, one for each state. What I think of is a great sandwich, maybe slices of roast turkey, grilled chicken, or lean roast beef. Tuna packed in water is also good.

Bring all your supplies to work on Monday. When lunch rolls around, pack your fillings of choice between slices of whole-grain bread. Apply mustard or low-cal mayo. Add all the tomato, lettuce, pickle, salsa, olives, relish, salt, or pepper that you desire. (Use plenty of onion if you aren't planning a one-on-one with the boss in the afternoon!) Add salad or soup, and you've got the perfect all-American lunch.

My friend David buys a 6-pound turkey breast when it's on sale. He cooks it on Sunday, has it hot for dinner that night, and has enough left over for another dinner and 2 or 3 lunches at the office.

Also, don't forget those batch meals you prepared over the weekend. An individual-size portion in a plastic container, heated in the office microwave, makes a delicious lunch. Shake things up for variety. Have hot batch lunches on Monday, Wednesday, and Friday, and cold sandwiches on Tuesday and Thursday. Or, heck, do the reverse: It's your choice!

BOTTOM LINE: Lose 22–30 pounds

Substituting an all-American lunch for burgers and fries will save you 300–400 calories a day.

> **IT SOUNDS** elementary, but batch cooking and calorie control won't work unless you know how much to buy ahead of time.

■ ORGANIZED SHOPPING ensures that your larder is always full of nutritious, easy-to-prepare foods. But this approach only works if you know how much to buy for the coming week.

If you've planned to eat 3 servings of your favorite fruit every day, for example, you have to get 21 portions (assuming you're the only one eating it). Some of that can be fresh, some canned, some frozen—but you have to be sure you come home with 21 portions.

On my last shopping trip, I bought 2 pounds of frozen blueberries so I could have a half cup each morning with my cereal. I also bought enough orange juice so that my significant other, Jack, and I could each have 6 ounces every morning.

Using the same sort of calculation, I bought 14 peaches, 14 plums, and 14 nectarines (one a day for each of us), along with 2 quarts of blackberries (Jack has them with his cereal, and I enjoy them as an occasional treat). You get the idea.

Don't forget: Get all the ingredients you need to prepare two large batch recipes for the week.

BOTTOM LINE: Lose 20–80 pounds

Knowing exactly how much you need to buy guarantees that you won't run out of key ingredients during the week. Which means you'll be less likely to make a last-minute run to the fast-food takeout line.

> **I DON'T KNOW** about you, but I'm often rushed in the mornings. The only way I'll eat a nutritionally sound breakfast is to have an ample supply of ready-to-go foods.

■ WHEN you make your weekly trip to the grocery store, be certain that you get enough breakfast essentials. You don't want any excuses for skipping breakfast, or stopping at a fast-food outlet on your way to work.

First, you have to decide what you like to eat. That's pretty simple for me: I love oatmeal! When I make my grocery list, I make sure I'll have enough of everything. I usually buy a large container of old-fashioned rolled oats, a gallon of milk, a pound of nuts, a box of brown sugar, a stick of light butter, and a quart of blueberries (or raspberries, just for a change). I also get a jar of toasted wheat germ and a quart of my favorite, fresh-squeezed orange juice.

Incidentally, I buy fresh blueberries in season. The rest of the year, frozen is fine.

BOTTOM LINE: Lose 21 pounds

The great thing about my oatmeal breakfast is that I feel full and satisfied all morning—no need for a vending machine snack. Most important, I don't have cravings that send me to a restaurant for lunch. I'm able to enjoy the simple—but delicious—lunches I've planned. My guess is that starting the day with a healthful breakfast saves me at least 200 calories a day!

#153 *defrost the freezer*

YOU WANT to make room for delicious frozen meals. My freezer is always full, which means I don't have to rush out for fast food when I'm hungry. My freezer is a fast-food outlet.

■ FORGET all the nasty things you've heard about frozen foods. Today's supermarkets stock hundreds of items that are nutritious as well as low in calories. Many of today's frozen foods taste pretty darn good, too.

When buying frozen foods, check the number of calories on the nutrition label. I eat meals with 500 calories or less. Jack, on the other hand, needs about 700 calories per meal. He selects dishes accordingly. If a frozen dinner doesn't include vegetables, I'll buy some frozen vegetable or fresh produce to go with the main dish.

The selection of frozen foods is enormous. I love a macaroni and cheese meal every so often, as well as meatloaf and mashed potatoes, french fries, pizza, and sometimes Thai or Indian food. You'll find most of these at any time in my freezer.

BOTTOM LINE: Lose 18–51 pounds

Stocking up on delicious, wholesome frozen dinners can save you 300–500 calories per dinner—even more if you really go wild when you find yourself at a takeout window. Eat healthful frozen meals four nights a week and you'll drop a minimum of 18 pounds. Eat them more often—and reduce your consumption of rich snacks or restaurant food at the same time—and you'll lose a lot more.

> **WANT to eat at the best restaurants in town? Go for it! Just don't break the "calorie bank" by doing it every night.**

■ I LOVE going to a fine restaurant and indulging in whatever my heart desires. My particular favorite: Sitting at the "chef's table" with one of the top chefs in the city taking care of my every whim. Of course, I plan an event like this with some care.

First things first. You can go to excellent restaurants regularly and still lose weight. Even though the food might be swimming in butter or cream sauce, you're not eating it all the time. Life is short. Enjoy.

For many of us, however, restaurants are a fallback from bad planning. We eat out when we're too tired at the end of the day to cook, or when there's nothing in the refrigerator. Do this a lot, and you're going to gain weight.

Personally, I've found that my body can cope nicely if I limit my restaurant indulgences to once a week. Others might be able to do it 2 or even 3 times without negative repercussions.

I do advise ordering simply most of the time. Save the real splurges for special occasions, or at least "thank God it's Friday" celebrations.

BOTTOM LINE: Lose 20–30 pounds

Go to a restaurant 3 times a week instead of your usual 5, and you'll save about 500 calories each evening. Heck, be radical—only go once a week. You'll save 2,000 calories!

10
Mix and Match to Lose Whatever You Want

I n this chapter, I've arranged all of the strategies in *Diet Simple* by pounds. It's designed so you can mix and match your own tips. The beauty of *Diet Simple* is that it's painless. Start by analyzing your normal eating routine, and look over the strategies outlined in the previous 154 tips. Look for changes that are simple enough for you to live with. Your personality and preferences should dictate what you decide—not some stringent diet police dictating your plan.

Then, start perusing the "Lose 2 to 5 Pounds" category, which follows. Are there a few painless techniques you can try that would be a snap to do? How about "doing a hunger check" or "choosing surf over turf?" Next, peruse the "Lose 6 to 10 Pounds" strategies. Would it be simple for you to "eat before you party," or "mine-sweep for calorie bombs?"

I tell everyone—those who are very overweight as well as those who simply want to drop a few pounds—that it makes more sense to set modest initial goals, and to achieve those goals by tinkering with, rather than completely overhauling, their diets and lifestyles. Drastic diets can certainly result in impressive weight loss, but they're not healthy, and no one sticks with them very long. I'd rather see people set reasonable goals and achieve them than shoot for the moon and fail completely.

Losing 10 pounds in two months is a great first goal. For some people, that's all they'll need to lose in order to feel better—and to fit into some of those closes that are hanging in the back of the closet! For those who need to lose more, setting an initial 10-pound goal makes the entire process less daunting. I've seen the excitement build as the pounds come off a little bit each week. People start getting giddy as they approach the 10-pound mark—and by the time they reach it, they're almost always eager to keep going.

Nearly everyone can lose a pound a week. Losing a total of 10 pounds in two months, for instance, is easier than most people imagine.

Then, take a look at the higher weight loss categories, where the strategies may be slightly more challenging. In the "Lose 16 to 20 Pounds" category, are you ready to "buy better dairy," "eat more to eat less," or "turn on your VCR?" Only you can decide what you're ready for.

In all, choose several tips from each category. Find the ones that fit your lifestyle, that you would actually enjoy doing. Mix and match to decide how much you want to lose. Be creative. Make sure the tips fit your personality. And have fun.

LOSE 2 TO 5 POUNDS		
TIP #	**TIP**	**LBS.**
#6	baked not fried	3
#12	hold the tuna salad	3–6
#14	choose "surf"	4–18
#17	add the whipped cream	3–16
#27	eat more pizza	3–6
#33	reduce noise pollution	5
#68	say "no" to something bad	5–15
#69	say "yes" to something good	5–15
#76	score the best real estate	4
#90	have a flying picnic	3
#96	be a "shopping tourist"	5
#97	the briefcase surprise	5
#98	the "first lady" technique	4–6
#112	learn to count	4–7
#113	think active thoughts	4
#114	park the car	2
#115	be a culture vulture	3
#116	dance!	3–6
#117	look for home grown	3
#118	the amazing cooler	5
#120	drop food hints	4
#121	compliment lavishly	4
#122	stretch	2–3
#124	drown yourself	4–21
#127	read the fine print	4–10
#129	naked salad	2–16
#132	break the rules	4–20
#135	start with salad	3–35
#136	do a hunger check	3–49

LOSE 6 TO 10 POUNDS		
TIP #	TIP	LBS.
#1	the sundae solution	9–35
#2	set your alarm	6–14
#4	do the bed stretch	7
#8	"pedal" while you prattle	10–42
#11	eat more slowly	10
#13	say "no" to pushers	13
#16	eat, then shop	9
#20	minesweep for calorie bombs	10–29
#21	beware the burger blast	6–16
#25	cook with spray	10–31
#30	lose with tailoring	9
#32	join Martha Stewart	9
#45	walk somewhere…anywhere	6–14
#51	dream	10
#60	kiss your spouse	7
#72	the 25 percent blowout	9
#74	eat before you party	7
#75	the 30-second rule	7
#78	imagine every move	6
#79	give away leftovers	7
#81	think exercise	6–14
#82	serve…pause…serve	7–14
#83	bring out the produce	10–21
#84	be a lousy host	7–15
#87	start a trend	6–7
#88	shift your appetite clock	9
#89	win with first class	7
#91	terminal snacks	7
#92	steal a gym	9

LOSE 6 TO 10 POUNDS (CON'T)		
TIP #	**TIP**	**LBS.**
#93	luggage calisthenics	9
#99	join the snack committee	9–17
#103	make faces	6
#104	lose the minibar key	8
#105	get elastic	6
#106	bring your exercise instructor	10
#107	portable yogis	7
#108	heat up the day	7
#109	call home	7
#110	travel with your hobby	7
#111	plan your dream house	7
#123	watch out for calorie creep	7–37
#125	eat simple breakfasts	6–30
#128	words count	8–40
#130	eat plenty of filet	7–70
#131	the power of doggie bags	6–49
#134	irritate the waiter	6–42
#145	hamburgers without end	6–18
#147	the secret is plastics	10–40
#149	slash corporate calories	6–18

LOSE 11 TO 15 POUNDS		
TIP #	TIP	LBS.
#10	substitute oil for butter	12
#18	take up yoga	13
#19	less creamy, more oily	13
#22	take center stage	12
#39	say "hi" to your feet	11–22
#40	win with gadgets	12–52
#56	don't go home	15–30
#61	breathe, bathe, relax	15
#86	the chocolate cardiac challenge	15
#94	pretend you're still home	14
#95	harass the hotel	14
#119	rest-stop workouts	15
#133	have a "premeal"	15–75
#146	eat your office supplies	11–60

LOSE 16 TO 20 POUNDS		
TIP #	TIP	LBS.
#5	pour another glass	17–22
#7	think positive thoughts	20–30
#15	tighten a muscle	19
#23	the dilution solution	18
#26	the "whole" story	21
#31	splurge on expensive delicacies	17
#38	buy better dairy	16
#41	breathe deeply	17
#42	more snacking, fewer calories	19–26
#43	turn on your VCR	16–66
#48	eat by the clock	20–80
#53	get sexy lingerie	18
#80	prioritize	16
#137	shop by the book	20–80
#139	the joy of index cards	20–80
#143	save time with frozen produce	20–50
#144	eat more to eat less	20–50
#148	shop online	20–80
#151	learn to count	20–80
#152	take breakfast shortcuts	21
#153	defrost the freezer	18–51
#154	do some fine dining	20–30

LOSE 21 TO 25 POUNDS		
TIP #	**TIP**	**LBS.**
#24	muffin madness	21–52
#35	the amazing sandwich	21
#37	lead a snake dance	24
#44	listen when you chew	21
#46	write it and lose it	23
#54	listen to the Eagles	21
#57	eat early	22–30
#62	love your pet	22
#63	light a candle	21
#77	savor each bite	21
#85	lighten up	21
#126	fish for health	22
#140	coffee ain't enough	22–30
#141	eat breakfast at work	22–30
#150	eat all-American	22–30

LOSE 26 TO 30 POUNDS		
TIP #	**TIP**	**LBS.**
#29	steal a TV	27
#36	hit the ground running	28–42
#47	fight the beast	30
#49	confront your feelings	26
#52	do some calorie shifting	30
#55	late snack	30
#59	sing in the shower	26–31
#64	get moving fast	30–54
#66	eat a brownie every Friday	30
#142	cook more than you can eat	30–42

LOSE 31 TO 35 POUNDS		
TIP #	TIP	LBS.
#50	let yourself live	31–46
#58	satisfy your sweet tooth	34
#65	examine your goals	31
#67	learn from mistakes	31
#70	"happy hour" at home	33
#71	start a social club	33
#73	only eat the best	31
#100	the happy-hour trap	31
#101	better than beer nuts	31
#102	work out, then eat out	35

LOSE 36-PLUS POUNDS		
TIP #	TIP	LBS.
#3	walk the dog	46–88
#9	eat more salads	36
#28	shop at the farmers' market	36
#34	march for a cause	60
#138	don't cook on weekdays	36

Part 3
Fast and Delicious
batch recipes
from the best chefs

N o matter how many pounds you're looking to lose, or what tips you choose to get you there, Batch Cooking is an integral part of *Diet Simple*. Make these recipes on the weekend, and you have great dinners ready to go on Tuesday, Thursday, and Saturday nights. Just knowing that you have delicious meals ready to go in minutes will keep you away from high-calorie, disorganized eating. Plus, Batch Cooking saves you time and money and nurtures your spirit all at once.

I recommend the following stew and soup recipes because they're delicious and satisfying. You won't go hungry. They're perfect for the chilly seasons—when most people's taste buds sway toward the hearty. And the Main Dish Salads are perfect calorie reducers for warmer months. Try some or all. The flavors will bring you culinary ecstasy!

The French Culinary Institute's Veal Stew with Carrots, La Boutarde

THIS VEAL STEW IS THE PERFECT meal for a brisk fall or winter day. The aromas will fill your home with warmth and comfort. This is also a very simple recipe. The preparation is fast, but I add an hour to the cooking time because I double the vegetables and the Herbes de Provence. I also use wine only (no water). The beauty of this recipe is that the measurements are not precise. You can cook to your own taste.

The veal rump can be found at a butcher's or a specialty market, if you can't find it at your grocery store. A substitute would be veal shoulder, which is typically used for stews, but is not as lean as the rump. If you're on a budget, beef round is an excellent—and very lean—substitute.

Ingredients

4 servings

- 1 tablespoon olive oil
- 2 pounds veal rump, well-trimmed and cut into 2-inch cubes salt and freshly ground white pepper
- 2 medium carrots, cut into ½-inch slices
- 1 medium onion, chopped
- 1½ cups dry white wine
- 1 cup water
- 2 medium very ripe tomatoes, peeled, cored, seeded, and chopped
- 2 teaspoons Herbes de Provence*
- 1 bay leaf
- 3 small all-purpose potatoes, peeled and quartered

Directions

- Warm the oil in a large sauté pan over medium-high heat. When hot, add no more than half the veal and sear for 3 minutes, or until the veal has evenly browned on all sides. Do not crowd the pan or scorch the meat. Using a slotted spoon, transfer the veal to a Dutch oven. Continue searing the veal until all of the meat has been browned. Season with salt and pepper.

■ In the same pan over medium heat, sauté the carrots and onions for 3 minutes, or until the onions are translucent. Reduce the heat and stir in the wine. Using a wooden spoon, stir vigorously to lift the browned bits from the bottom of the pan.

■ Pour into the Dutch oven. Add the water, tomatoes, Herbes de Provence, and bay leaf.

■ Place the Dutch oven over medium heat and bring the stew to a boil. Reduce the heat to medium-low, cover, and simmer for one hour.

■ Add the potatoes and simmer for 35 minutes, or until the potatoes are tender.

■ Taste and adjust the seasoning. Remove and discard the bay leaf.

Chef's Note: Herbes de Provence is a mixture of dried herbs that often includes basil, lavender, rosemary, sage, thyme, and others. Look for it in the spice section of your supermarket.

Per Serving

calories 437
total fat 12g
saturated fat 4g

total carbohydrate 22g
dietary fiber 4g
protein 60g

"Veal Stew with Carrots, La Boutarde" originally appeared in **The French Culinary Institute's Salute to Healthy Cooking**, *by Alain Sailhac, Jacques Pépin, André Soltner, Jacques Torres, and the Faculty of the French Culinary Institute.*
© 1998 The French Culinary Institute.

Graham Kerr's Turkey Pot Pie *pie*

THIS IS A LIGHTER take on the traditional American comfort food. The dish is basically a flavorful turkey stew in a creamy sauce topped with savory cheese biscuits. It's delicious with all of its flavors and textures, the strong, crunchy turnips balanced by the sweet parsnips. This saves beautifully in the refrigerator for lunches at the office or midweek dinners.

4 servings

Ingredients

1 teaspoon nonaromatic olive oil

½ sweet onion, cut in ¼-inch pieces and diced (1 cup)

2 turnips, peeled and cut in ½-inch pieces

2 small parsnips, peeled and cut in ½ inch pieces (½ cup)

1½ cups homemade turkey or low sodium chicken stock

¼ teaspoon salt

⅛ teaspoon pepper

1 pound broccoli

2½ cups cooked turkey

Sauce:

¾ pounds parsnips, peeled, roughly chopped, and steamed until tender

1 cup evaporated skim milk

¼ teaspoon salt

Cheese Biscuits (adapted from *Eating Well—Secrets of Low-Fat Cooking*):

1 cup all-purpose flour

1 cup cake flour

1 tablespoon sugar

1½ teaspoons baking powder

½ teaspoon baking soda

¼ teaspoon salt

1½ teaspoons cold, hard, butter-flavored margarine, cut into small pieces

¾ cup buttermilk

1 tablespoon nonaromatic olive oil

¼ cup grated low-fat sharp cheddar cheese

1 tablespoon low-fat milk to brush on top

Directions

- Heat the oil in a chef's pan or skillet on medium high, sauté the onions, carrots, turnips, and parsnips on medium heat 3 minutes. Pour in the stock and season with salt and pepper. Bring to a boil, reduce the heat, cover and simmer until the vegetables are tender, 6 minutes.

- Whiz the steamed parsnips in a blender with a little of the evaporated milk until smooth and velvety, another 30 seconds.

Biscuits:

- Preheat the oven to 425 degrees. Coat a baking sheet with oil spray. Whisk together the flours, sugar, baking powder, soda, and salt in a bowl or combine in a processor.

- Scatter the pieces of margarine over the top and cut in with 2 knives or pulse 2–3 times in a processor. Make a well in the center of the dry ingredients and pour in the buttermilk and oil. Stir with a fork until just blended or pulse 2–3 times in a processor.

- Knead the dough very lightly on a floured board. Pat or roll out about ½ inch thick and cut into 4 large (3½-inch) biscuits. Place on the prepared baking sheet, brush with milk, dust with cheese, and bake 15 minutes or until golden.

- While the biscuits are baking, lay the broccoli on the simmering vegetables and cook 6 minutes or until tender but still bright green. Stir in the turkey and parsnip sauce and heat through.

- Biscuits by the nature of their chemistry are high in calories and fat. To reduce the risk, make a whole recipe, cut the tops off 4 to use in the recipe, and save the bottoms and extra biscuit to toast for breakfast.

To serve:

- Spoon the turkey mixture into 4 hot soup plates and lay the biscuit halves on top.

Per Serving

calories 438	total carbohydrate 51g
total fat 9g	dietary fiber 5g
saturated fat 2g	protein 38g

Graham Kerr is an internationally known culinary consultant, television personality, award-winning author, and colorful motivational speaker. His focus is on serving people who want to make healthy, creative lifestyle changes and he believes that the only lasting changes are the ones that we enjoy. He is the star of his own PBS series, The Gathering Place, Where the Pan Sizzles and Science Smiles.

Jacques Pépin's "Poule Au Pot"

POULE AU POT IS A RICH, aromatic, easy-to-prepare main-course meal in one pot. The dish, according to Pépin, originated in the sixteenth century under the rule of Henry IV. But Pépin lightens the stew by removing the fat from the chicken stock. The French make the most flavorful stocks, and cloves is one of their secret ingredients. Combined with thyme, rosemary, and bay leaves, this creates a surprisingly fresh and savory flavor. Store in your refrigerator and pack in plastic containers for meals at the office.

4-6 servings

Ingredients

1 chicken (about 3½ pounds)
4 quarts water
1 teaspoon dried thyme leaves
1 teaspoon dried rosemary
3 bay leaves
12 cloves
2 teaspoon salt
1 teaspoon black
  peppercorns

Garnishes

16 slices from a bagette (2 ounce total), toasted in the oven
½ cup grated gruyere cheese
cornichons
hot mustard

Vegetables

2 large leeks (about 12 ounce total), cleaned
4 medium onions (10 ounce total), peeled
4 carrots (about 1 pound), peeled
1 small butternut squash (1 pound), peeled, seeded, and quartered
1 small savoy cabbage (about 1 pound), quartered
4 large mushrooms (about 4 ounces)

Directions

- Place the chicken, breast side down, with the neck and heart in a narrow stainless steel stockpot. Add the water, and bring it to a boil over high heat. Reduce the heat, and boil gently for 10 minutes. Skim the cooking liquid to remove the fat and impurities that come to the surface.
- Add the thyme, rosemary, bay leaves, cloves, salt, and peppercorns to the stock. Cover, and continue boiling gently for another 25 minutes. Remove the chicken from the pot; save the stock. When the chicken is cool enough to handle, pull off and discard the skin. Pull the meat from the bones, keeping it in the largest possible pieces. Set the meat aside, covered, in about ½ cup of the stock. Place the bones back in the remaining stock, and boil gently for another hour.
- Strain the stock twice through a strainer lined with paper towels. Rinse out the pot and return the stock to the pot. (You should have 8 to 9 cups. If necessary, adjust with water.)*

*This procedure should remove much of the fat. But if you have time, you could chill the stock until the remaining fat solidifies on top. Once it hardens, it's easy to remove and discard so that you have a fat-free stock.

For the vegetables
- Add the leeks, onions, carrots, squash, and cabbage to the stock, and bring to a boil, covered, for 15 minutes. Add the mushrooms and cook for another 5 minutes.
- Reheat the meat and the surrounding liquid, and arrange the meat in the center of a large platter. Remove the vegetables with a slotted spoon and arrange them around

the chicken. Ladle some of the stock into 4 to 6 small bowls, and serve it with the baguette slices and cheese. Pass around the cornichons and hot mustard at the table.

Per Serving

calories 402	total carbohydrate 40g
total fat 9.4g	dietary fiber 8g
saturated fat 3.5g	protein 42g

Jacques Pépin is a master chef, author, and teacher to a generation of famous chefs—as well as millions of enthusiastic home chefs. One of America's best-known cooking teachers, Pépin has published 19 books and numerous articles and has hosted acclaimed television cooking shows. His newest ventures include a two-hour public television special, Chez Pépin, celebrating his 50 years in the kitchen.

"Poule Au Pot" (Chicken Stew) is from *Jacques Pépin's Table: The Complete Today's Gourmet*.

© *Jacques Pépin*

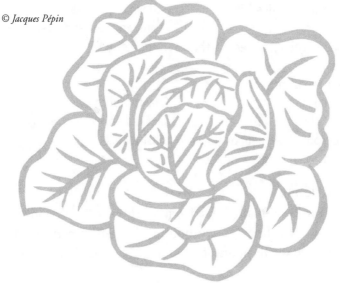

John Ash's Grandmother's Pot Roast

CHEF JOHN ASH SAYS his grandmother had a real touch for wholesome, comfort foods like this savory pot roast. The meat is cooked until falling off the bone, *stracotto,* as it would be called in Italy. Styles may change; dishes like this won't. That's why I decided to include it in *Diet Simple*. It's lean and a great source of protein, iron and vitamin A. You can keep it in your refrigerator for up to three days and slice it for a sandwich or toss it in a salad using Dan Puzo's Red Wine Vinaigrette (page 275).

6–8 servings

Ingredients

3 pounds tri-tip or bottom round of beef

salt and freshly ground black pepper

4 tablespoons olive oil

3 cups sliced onions

1 cup leeks, sliced into rounds

1½ cups celery, sliced on the bias

1½ cups carrots, cut in wedges

¼ cup slivered garlic

¼ teaspoon red pepper flakes

4 cups hearty red wine

3 cups rich beef stock

2 cups seeded and diced tomatoes

2 large bay leaves

1 teaspoon fennel seed

2 teaspoons *each* minced fresh thyme, sage, and oregano leaves (1 teaspoon *each* dried)

Garnish:
Roasted potatoes and sautéed shiitake or wild mushrooms

Directions

- Trim beef of all visible fat and season with salt and pepper. In a large, heavy bottomed roasting pan, quickly brown the meat on all sides in the olive oil. Remove meat and add the onions, leeks, celery, carrots, and garlic and cook over moderate heat until vegetables just begin to color and onions are translucent.

- Return meat to the pan and add pepper flakes, red wine, stock, tomatoes, and herbs. Bring to a simmer, cover, and place in a preheated 375 degree oven for 2 to 2½ hours, or until meat is very tender and almost falling apart.
- Strain the liquid from the meat and vegetables. Allow the liquid to sit for a few minutes so that the fat will rise to the surface. Strain off and discard fat. Return the liquid to the pan and, over high heat, reduce by approximately ⅓ to concentrate flavors (if desired, thicken with 2 teaspoons cornstarch dissolved in wine or water). Correct seasoning with salt and pepper.
- Return meat and braising vegetables to pan and warm through. Slice meat and arrange in shallow bowls along with some of the braising vegetables. Generously ladle reduced sauce around and garnish with roasted potatoes and mushrooms.

Per Serving

calories 430	total carbohydrate 16g
total fat 14g	dietary fiber 3g
saturated fat 4g	protein 40g

John Ash established his restaurant, John Ash & Company, in Northern California's wine country in 1980. Soon, he was selected by Food & Wine *magazine as one of America's "hot new chefs." The restaurant has regularly been recognized as one of America's best by leading critics. He has written an award-winning cookbook,* From the Earth to the Table: John Ash's Wine Country Cuisine *(Dutton).*

Kaz Sushi Bistro's Asian Vegetable Noodles

THIS IS A PERFECT basic stir-fry recipe for great batch meals. You can use any number of vegetables or meats. Add one pound of shrimp, chicken breast, or tofu, and you have a complete dinner. Try a variety of fresh vegetables—just about any will do. The aroma of the sesame oil, ginger, garlic, and soy sauce will make you feel like a genuine Asian cook.

4 servings

Ingredients

½ pound vermicelli noodles or rice

1 tablespoon vegetable oil

½ Spanish onion, julienne

½ red bell pepper, julienne

5 dried shiitake mushrooms (or any type of fresh), julienne

½ carrot, shredded

1 bunch scallions, julienne

¼ cup soy sauce

1½ tablespoons sugar

black pepper

4 tablespoons sesame oil

1 teaspoon ginger, grated (optional)

1 teaspoon garlic, minced (optional)

Directions

- Soak dried shiitake in warm water until soft (about one hour), if not using fresh shiitake mushrooms. Cut all vegetables.
- Cook noodles in boiling water for 5 minutes, drain, and toss with 1 tablespoon of the sesame oil, set aside.
- Sauté onion, ginger, and garlic in pan with the vegetable oil until soft. Then add carrot, shiitake, red bell pepper, and scallion with soy sauce and sugar.

- Add noodles into the pan, toss with the vegetables, and add the remaining 3 tablespoons of the sesame oil and black pepper

Chef's Note: sesame oil adds a rich flavor but loses some of the flavor in cooking. This is why vegetable oil is used for the vegetable sauté and sesame oil is saved for the tossing.

Per Serving

calories 440	total carbohydrate 61g
total fat 18g	dietary fiber 5g
saturated fat 2.5g	protein 10g

KAZ Sushi Bistro's chef-owner **Kazuhiro Okochi** *(Kaz) was the first to introduce an original new concept—"Free Style Japanese Cuisine." "My goal," says Kaz, "is to create simple and authentic Japanese cuisine as well as innovative dishes with a Western touch." The Washington, D.C., Bistro has garnered many awards, including Highest Rated Sushi Bar by the* Zagat Survey 2001.

Nora Pouillon's Ratatouille

RATATOUILLE IS AN AUTHENTIC Provençal ragout of onions, eggplants, peppers, zucchini, and tomatoes, stewed slowly in olive oil and flavored with garlic and fresh herbs. Cutting up the vegetables is time consuming, so I like to make double the amount and use the leftovers...

- at room temperature the next day with grilled chicken or fish;
- mixed with eggs and cheese for a quiche;
- heated and stirred with beaten eggs, spiced with chilis, and served with sliced ham, Proscuitto, or cooked lean sausage as Piperade or Basque dish;
- reheated and used as sauce for freshly cooked pasta, garnished with feta or goat cheese, with the addition of pitted black olives;
- as minestrone, heated with vegetable or chicken stock, adding a can of drained cannellini beans and maybe a spoon of pesto on top.

The trick of a good ratatouille is not to overcook the vegetables. They have to be added one after the other, depending on the amount of time they need to cook to be just tender.

6–8 servings

Ingredients

½ cup olive oil
1 large onion, chopped
1 tablespoon garlic, minced
1–2 eggplants (2 pounds) cut into 1-inch cubes

2 peppers, red, green, or yellow, cut into 1-inch squares
2 zucchini (1½ pounds) cut into 1-inch cubes
1.5 pounds tomatoes, peeled and cut into 1-inch cubes

Ingredients (cont'd)

salt and freshly ground
black pepper
1 tablespoon fresh thyme,
minced

½ tablespoon fresh
rosemary, minced
2 tablespoons fresh parsley
or basil, minced

Directions

- Heat olive oil in a large skillet until hot.
- Add the onions and stew for 10 minutes until soft. Add the garlic, then the eggplants and peppers. Cover and cook slowly for 20 minutes.
- Add the zucchini, cook for 5 minutes, then, last, add the tomatoes and cook for an additional 5 minutes or less.
- Season with salt and pepper and the minced herbs.

Per Serving

calories 220	total carbohydrate 18g
total fat 16g	dietary fiber 6g
saturated fat 2g	protein 3g

Nora Pouillon is the chef and owner of two of Washington, D.C.'s, most popular restaurants. Featuring organic, multi-ethnic cuisine, the internationally known Restaurant Nora opened in 1979 and has been praised for its delicious, high-quality food and healthy approach to eating. In 1999, Nora became the first certified organic restaurant in the country. Nora received the 4-star rating from Mobile Travel Guide 2000 *and was voted one of the "Top 10 Healthiest Restaurants" by* Health *magazine.*

Phyllis Frucht's Chicken Lentil-Curry Stew

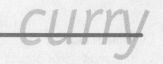

THIS RECIPE is one of the quickest and easiest batch recipes to make—about 20 minutes to prepare and 20 minutes to cook. Yet it's one of the most aromatic and elegant dinners you'll have. One chef I know gives this savory stew with an Indian flair a "3-D rating" for *delightful, delectable,* and *delicious!* Even though the okra is optional, I say "go for it."

The recipe may be prepared a day ahead, and it freezes well, too. To save time, use a large package of your favorite frozen vegetable blend. For a heartier meal, add cooked brown rice. Leaving the bones in the chicken thighs improves the stock and the flavor.

Ingredients

8 servings

- 1 tablespoon vegetable oil
- 2 pounds chicken thighs without skin
- 2 garlic cloves, minced
- 1 medium onion, peeled and minced
- 1 14.5 ounce can tomatoes, chopped
- 2 carrots, peeled and cut in ½-inch cubes
- 1 pound potatoes, peeled and cut in ¾ inch cubes
- ¾ pounds okra, sliced (optional)
- 1 pound dry lentils
- 4 cups water
- 2 tablespoons curry powder
- salt and pepper to taste
- 2 tablespoons cilantro, chopped (optional)

Directions

- Heat the oil in a 5-quart saucepan with a tight fitting lid. Season the chicken with salt and pepper. Fry until golden brown in the vegetable oil, a few minutes on each side.

Remove from the pan. Sauté the garlic and onions in the same pan, scraping up bits from the bottom of the pan, until soft and golden.

■ Add the vegetables and mix to coat well. Add the lentils, chicken, water, and seasonings, except for the cilantro. Bring to a boil and lower the flame. Cover and simmer for about 20 minutes until the potatoes and lentils are soft.

■ Sprinkle with cilantro and serve.

Per Serving

calories 370	total carbohydrate 49g
total fat 8g	dietary fiber 15g
saturated fat 2g	protein 29g

Phyllis Frucht is a chef and a teacher specializing in international cuisine from the Orient to India, Europe, the Middle East, and the Caribbean. She gives instruction in Washington, D.C., in elegant hands-on classes that include generous samplings of the foods with matching beverages and wine. Her menus often reflect the fusion of cross-cultural traditions and flavors.

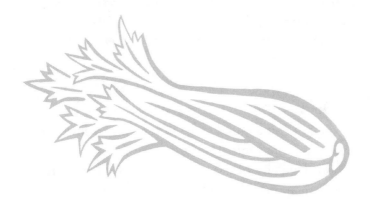

Tallmadge's Chili Non-Carne *chili*

I LOVE THIS SIMPLE, quick chili recipe. Of course, there're zillions of ways to make chili, but this recipe is easy to follow and it's meatless. And believe me, you won't miss the meat. This batch is packed with flavor. Use however much garlic or chili powder that appeals to you. I like mine hot and spicy!

I usually double the recipe so I have plenty for the week. This dish makes a great lunch or dinner alongside a green salad. I also serve it at parties as a dip next to fresh tomato salsa, light sour cream, and guacamole. It's perfect rolled up in a tortilla or stuffed in a taco with some cheese.

4 servings

Ingredients

1 tablespoon olive or canola oil
1 large onion, chopped
3 large garlic cloves, minced
3 tablespoons hot chili powder
1 large fresh green pepper, chopped
1 28-ounce can Italian plum tomatoes, chopped, including the liquid

1 pound can kidney or black beans, whichever is preferred
½ cup water or bouillon (to hydrate the bulgur)
½ cup bulgur (cracked wheat)
2 seeded jalapeno peppers, chopped, if desired
salt and pepper to taste

Directions

- Sauté the onions and garlic in the oil over low heat in a large pot until soft, 15 or more minutes.
- Add the chili powder and simmer for a few more minutes. Then add the fresh green pepper and cook until al

dente. Meanwhile, soak the bulgur in the boiling water for 15 minutes.

- Add all remaining ingredients including the bulgur and simmer slowly over low to medium heat until flavors are well blended and vegetables are cooked to the desired consistency.

- Adjust seasonings to your preference. Since many canned items were used, additional salt will probably not be needed.

Per Serving

calories 320	total carbohydrate 60g
total fat 7g	dietary fiber 14g
saturated fat 1g	protein 12g

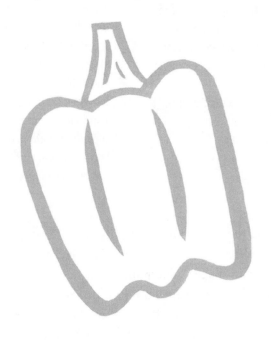

Xiomara's Arroz con Pollo *pollo*

THIS CREAMY, FILLING, and luxurious one-pot meal is rich enough to serve to guests, but it's deceivingly light (just don't tell the party; it'll spoil their fun). The pungent garlic and oregano combined with the tart juice and beer will transport you to the smells and sounds of Cuba. And it tastes even better the next day, which makes it a perfect batch recipe.

Ingredients

6–8 servings

8 garlic cloves peeled

1½ tablespoons salt

1 teaspoon black pepper

¼ cup fresh chopped oregano

¼ cup sour orange juice (or a 50/50 mix of sweet, fresh orange juice and fresh lime juice)

4 pounds skinned chicken thighs, and legs (with bones)

½ cup olive oil

2 medium red onions (peeled and finely chopped)

1 large red bell pepper, cored, seeded, and finely chopped

3 cups chicken broth (defatted)

6 strands saffron toasted in a dry skillet over medium heat for about 30 seconds, or until they lose their moisture

½ cup tomato sauce

2 cups short grain rice

2 bottles of beer

1 cup of frozen peas (thawed)

Directions

- Mash the garlic into paste with the salt and pepper.
- Add the garlic paste to the mixed citrus juice and pour over the chicken. Cover and refrigerate for about an hour.
- Heat the oil over medium heat in a wide shallow pan.
- Pour the marinade off of the chicken, and set the marinade aside. Blot the chicken before browning the pieces in the hot oil, and then set them aside.

- In the same oil, sauté the onions and red pepper until the onions are translucent, about 4 minutes. Add the broth, beer, saffron, oregano, tomato sauce, marinade, and the chicken and simmer for about 5 minutes. This a very moist dish. If needed add more beer or chicken broth.
- Add the rice and stir just enough to cover it with liquid. If the rice is not fully covered, add more broth or beer. Simmer uncovered, until all the liquid is absorbed and the rice is cooked, about 30 minutes. Add more broth or beer if needed.
- Remove pan from the heat and add peas five minutes before serving (the heat from the rice, will cook the peas), and mix.

Suggestions from Xiomara:
- "In my home, after cooking the chicken I debone just before serving. Cooking with the bones adds necessary flavor."
- "When cold, this dish may dry out a bit. Just add a cup chicken broth when reheating."

Per Serving

calories 540	total carbohydrate 52g
total fat 19g	dietary fiber 4g
saturated fat 3g	protein 33g

Xiomara Ardolina, chef-owner of Xiomara's in Pasadena, California, was born in Cuba and came to the United States at the age of 13. She established herself as one of the top restaurateurs in Southern California. In 1991, she opened Xiomara in Pasadena, featuring French cuisine. It was recognized as one of the finest restaurants in the Los Angeles area. In 1996, Xiomara began serving Nuevo Latino cuisine, and she's continued receiving high praise from the critics.

Tallmadge's White Beans with Garlic and Basil

I LOVE THESE BEANS. They taste deceptively rich, and they're easy to make. After I've made and stored a batch, I'll ladle a heap into a bowl and microwave for lunch, with a slice of whole-grain bread topped with smoked turkey, lean ham, or light cheese (or all three!) and some crunchy lettuce. Slice a spicy chicken sausage into a bowl, top with the beans, and pop in the microwave. Add a green salad and tart dressing and you've got a winning dinner. I usually double the recipe to have plenty during the week. Without meat, it will last more than a week refrigerated.

Ingredients

4 servings

½ pound dried small white (cannellini) beans, or 24 ounces canned rinsed beans
1 tablespoon olive oil
1½ onion, chopped
4 garlic cloves (more or less to taste—I double it)

1 quart defatted chicken stock
salt to taste
12 ounces (3 medium) fresh or canned tomatoes, drained, peeled, and chopped
1 large handful of fresh basil
juice from 1 lemon
freshly ground pepper

Directions

If you're using dried white beans

- Soak the beans in 1 quart of water overnight or up to 24 hours. Drain and rinse.
- Add 1 quart chicken stock to the beans along with 1 clove of garlic and ½ onion. Bring to a boil, reduce heat, cover,

and simmer 1½ hours or until the beans are almost tender. Add more water or stock to keep moist. Add salt to taste and finish cooking until beans are tender.

<u>Continue with your cooked dried beans or start here if you're using canned white beans</u>

■ Heat oil in a large, heavy soup pot or casserole and sauté the remaining onion and garlic over low to medium heat for 10 or 15 minutes or until soft.

■ Add the tomatoes, and more salt to taste and bring to a simmer. Simmer about 10 minutes then add the beans with their cooking liquid and simmer 15–20 minutes. If you used canned beans, rinse the beans then use enough stock to keep the beans moist while cooking.

■ At the end of the cooking time, add the fresh basil (it will get bitter if overcooked), fresh lemon juice, and freshly ground pepper. Mix together.

■ Let the beans sit at room temperature overnight to let the flavors blend.

■ Refrigerate and heat to serve.

Per Serving

calories 290   total carbohydrate 45g
total fat 4.5g   dietary fiber 16g
saturated fat 0.5g   protein 19g

Adapted from **Mediterranean Light**, *by Martha Rose Shulman (Bantam Books, 1989).*

Aquavit's Marcus Samuelsson's Corn Soup with Smoked Salmon

IF YOU LOVE CORN, this is the soup for you. Though corn is not a typically Swedish food, Chef Samuelsson uses it liberally here, combined with very typical Swedish ingredients—potatoes, salmon, tarragon, and sour cream. This soup uses the salmon bones to give the stock a depth of flavor to support the sweetness of the puréed corn and potatoes, but it can also be made without them. It is a delicious soup served warm or even at room temperature. You'll love it all week.

Ingredients

4 servings

6 ears of corn, shucked
6 fingerling or small new potatoes
2 tablespoons canola oil
Bones from 2 salmon (get these from your fish monger), optional
2 shallots, finely chopped
1 garlic clove, finely chopped
1 quart chicken stock

1 cup light sour cream, optional salt and freshly ground black pepper
2 sprigs fresh tarragon, finely chopped
2 sprigs fresh cilantro, finely chopped
6 ounces smoked salmon, cut into ½-inch cubes

Directions

- Preheat the oven to 400 degrees. Put the ears of corn and potatoes on a baking sheet and roast them for 25–30 minutes, until the potatoes are cooked through. Remove from the oven and let cool.

- Cut the corn kernels off the cobs and set them aside. Break each corn cob into 2 or 3 pieces and set aside. Peel the potatoes, and set aside.

- Put the canola oil in the bottom of a soup pot and turn the heat to medium high. Add the salmon bones, shallots, and garlic and sauté for about 3 minutes, until the shallots start to soften. Add the corn cobs and chicken stock and simmer for 30 minutes.

- Strain the stock, and combine it with the corn kernels and potatoes. Purée the soup in a blender, return it to the saucepan, and heat through over medium heat.

- When it's hot, turn off the heat, stir in the sour cream, and season to taste with salt and freshly ground black pepper.

- Garnish with tarragon and cilantro and top with cubes of smoked salmon.

Per Serving

Without Sour Cream	With Sour Cream
calories 470	calories 550
total fat 15g	total fat 20g
saturated fat 2g	saturated fat 6g
total carbohydrate 77g	total carbohydrate 81g
dietary fiber 5g	dietary fiber 5g
protein 19g	protein 23g

*Owner **Håkan Swahn's** goal with Aquavit, when he opened it in the heart of Manhattan in 1987, was to serve the finest Swedish cuisine available. And the restaurant has met with resounding success. Swahn and executive chef **Marcus Samuelsson** are basking in the glow of a 3-star review by the* New York Times, *and Marcus's 1999 James Beard Foundation award for best "Rising Star Chef."*

Border Grill's Turkey Albondigas Soup

WHAT COULD BE MORE hearty and inviting than a soup full of delicate meat balls and plenty of garlic, hot peppers, vegetables, and tomatoes. This dish is a spicy main course perfect on a cold day as it warms the soul. The Border Grill is renowned for serving zesty Latin street foods and this is a perfect example.

Ingredients

6 servings

- ¼ cup olive oil
- 8 garlic cloves, peeled
- 2 bunches cilantro, leaves only
- 1 tablespoon salt
- 1½ teaspoons freshly ground black pepper
- 1 pound ground turkey or chicken, preferably dark meat
- 1 large egg, beaten
- ⅔ cup fresh bread crumbs
- ⅓ cup vegetable oil
- 1 large leek, trimmed, washed, and thinly julienned
- 4 medium carrots, peeled and diced
- ¼ head white cabbage, cored and thinly sliced
- 1–2 jalapeno chilis, stemmed, seeded, and thinly julienned
- 3 medium Roma tomatoes, cored, seeded, and diced
- 2½ quarts chicken stock
- 3 tablespoons white vinegar

Directions

- Combine the olive oil, garlic, cilantro, and 1 teaspoon each of the salt and pepper in a blender. Purée until smooth.
- In a large bowl, mix together the turkey or chicken, egg, and cilantro paste. Add the bread crumbs and mix only until combined. Roll into small walnut-sized meatballs in the palms of your hands and place on a tray in the refrigerator.

- Heat 2 tablespoons of the vegetable oil in a large stockpot over high heat. Saute the leeks and carrots with the remaining 2 teaspoons salt and ½ teaspoon pepper for 2–4 minutes. Add the cabbage, jalapenos, and tomatoes and cook, stirring frequently, until the vegetables are limp, about 3 minutes longer. Pour in the chicken stock. Bring to a boil, reduce to a simmer, and cook, uncovered, 15 minutes.
- Meanwhile, heat the remaining oil in a medium skillet over medium heat until nearly smoking. Add the chilled meatballs in batches, shaking the pan to prevent sticking, and brown on all sides. Transfer with a slotted spoon to paper towels to drain.
- When all the meatballs are browned, transfer to the simmering stock and cook an additional 5–10 minutes. Stir in the vinegar and serve hot.

Per Serving

calories 460	total carbohydrate 28g
total fat 31g	dietary fiber 4g
saturated fat 7g	protein 20g

Mary Sue Milliken and *Susan Feniger, chef-owners of The Border Grill and Ciudad in Santa Monica, Los Angeles, and Las Vegas are the stars of the popular Television Food Network show* Too Hot Tamales. *Though they are multimedia figures of television and radio, have written cookbooks, and own several restaurants, the two never lose sight of the pleasure that cooking brings them.*

"Turkey Albondigas Soup" was reprinted from Mesa Mexicana, by Mary Sue Milliken and Susan Feniger, published by William Morrow ©1994.

Café des Artistes' Seafood Gazpacho, Sixty-Seventh Street Style

GAZPACHO EPITOMIZES the feeling of summer. When I purée my gazpacho, I leave it coarse and chunky. The garnish of fresh dill, scallions, cucumber, and croutons is essential to the soup's success. The added crunch and flavor go a long way to satisfy your senses. Adding shrimp to the gazpacho makes this a main course dish—one you can keep in your refrigerator for up to 3 days.

Ingredients

8-10 servings

2½ pounds red ripe tomatoes, peeled, seeded, and chopped

1 cup coarsely chopped Bermuda onion

½ cup each chopped green pepper and chopped carrot

1 clove of garlic, peeled

5 cups tomato juice

⅓ cup red wine vinegar

salt and freshly ground black pepper to taste

2 tablespoons olive oil

8 ounces tiny shrimp, shells removed, deveined, and lightly cooked

dash of Louisiana-type hot sauce

Garnish:

¼ cup chopped fresh dill

6 medium scallions, white part only, washed and cut into ¼-inch dice

1 large cucumber, peeled, seeded, and cut into ¼-inch dice

1 cup freshly toasted croutons

Directions

- Process tomatoes, onion, green pepper, carrot, and garlic in a food processor until the mixture takes on a rough texture.

- Stir in tomato juice and vinegar, and season with salt and pepper. Whisk in olive oil. Chill for at least 3 hours.
- Add shrimp. Adjust seasoning with hot sauce, and serve sprinkled with dill in chilled bowls, with crocks of scallion, cucumber, and croutons on the side.

Per Serving

calories 120	total carbohydrate 17g
total fat 4g	dietary fiber 3g
saturated fat 0.5g	protein 7g

* This dish is a great source of vitamins A and C.

*Since June 1991, **Thomas Ferlesch** has been the executive chef of the 3-star Café des Artistes, one of the 10 most popular restaurants in New York City, as ranked by the* Zagat *Survey 2000. The Café, owned and operated by Jenifer and George Lang, was named one of the "50 Best Restaurants in the United States" by* Conde Nast Traveler.

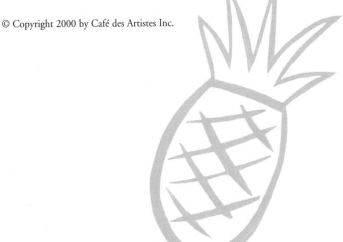

Judy Zeidler's Hearty and Versatile Vegetable Soup

VEGETABLE SOUPS ARE FAST and simple to make. They can be prepared in advance and stored in the refrigerator for a week or more until ready to serve. Most soups are even better the next day, and the longer they cook the more concentrated they become. Garnish this soup with chopped vegetables, sautéed mushrooms, or grilled onions.

Purée the leftover soup, and it can be used as a sauce for pasta on the second night and a sauce for fish on the third night (see the following recipes).

Ingredients

6 servings

¼ cup olive oil
2 medium leeks, finely diced
2 cloves garlic, minced
4 medium carrots, finely diced
4 stalks celery, finely diced
2 small new potatoes, unpeeled, finely diced
1 large zucchini, finely diced

¼ cup minced fresh parsley
6–8 cups water (or fat-free stock if preferred)
salt, to taste
freshly ground black pepper, to taste
2 tablespoons fresh basil, thinly sliced
freshly grated Parmesan cheese (optional)

Directions

- In a large heavy pot, heat olive oil over medium heat. Add leeks, garlic, carrots, celery, potatoes, zucchini, and parsley. Sauté 5 to 10 minutes, stirring until tender.

- Add water, bring to a boil over high heat, reduce heat and simmer, partially covered, for 30 minutes, stirring occasionally. Season with salt and pepper to taste.
- Add basil and simmer until vegetables are soft, about 15 minutes more. Ladle 1 cup of soup into blender and purée; return to soup and mix well.
- Ladle into heated soup bowls and sprinkle with grated Parmesan cheese.

Hearty Vegetable Soup with Sautéed Fish

6 servings

Ingredients

Hearty Vegetable Soup (see recipe)
1 pound salmon fillets or white fish

¼ cup Panko Crumbs or bread crumbs
¼ cup olive oil

Directions

- Place soup in a food processor and purée. Transfer to a saucepan and set aside.
- Dice the fish fillets into 1-inch cubes. Dip in Panko Crumbs and place on paper towels.
- Heat olive oil in a nonstick skillet and sauté prepared fish fillets on both sides until lightly brown. Transfer to paper towels until ready serve.
- To serve, heat the soup, ladle in heated bowls, and spoon the sauteed fish in the center.

Pasta with Vegetable Sauce

Ingredients

6 servings

2 cups puréed vegetable
soup (see recipe)

6 ounces dry spaghetti or
tagliatelli

Parmesan cheese

Directions

- In a large skillet heat the puréed soup. Bring a large pot of water to a boil and add spaghetti or tagliatelli. Cook until tender.
- Drain, add to the sauce, and toss to coat pasta. Serve in heated shallow bowls and sprinkle with Parmesan cheese.

Per Serving
Vegetable Soup
calories 160
total fat 9g
saturated fat 1.5g
total carbohydrate 19g
dietary fiber 4g
protein 3g

Per Serving
With Sautéed Fish
calories 400
total fat 27g

saturated fat 4g
total carbohydrate 22g
dietary fiber 4g
protein 18g

Per Serving With Fish and
Whole Wheat Pasta
calories 495
total fat 27g
saturated fat 4g
total carbohydrate 43g
dietary fiber 7g
protein 21g

Judy Zeidler is the author of the widely acclaimed The Gourmet Jewish Cook *as well as* Judy Zeidler's International Deli Cookbook, *among others. Her weekly syndicated television show,* Judy's Kitchen, *airs on the Jewish Television Network. Zeidler is a regular contributor to the* Los Angeles Times *and the* Jewish Journal.

Kjerstin's Simple Hot and Sour Soup

THIS RECIPE of my mother's is so irresistible that friends have told me they've finished off the whole batch in one evening. Use it as a first course or a main course.

Ingredients

4 servings

4 diced dry black (Shiitake) mushrooms or fresh mushrooms

5 cups chicken broth

1 chicken breast

¼ cup bamboo shoots, slivered

½ cup rice wine vinegar

2 tablespoons soy sauce

1–2 green onions, cut into 2-inch slivers

1 tablespoon finely chopped cilantro

1 teaspoon Tabasco sauce

½ teaspoon pepper

3 tablespoons cornstarch

¼ cup water

1 egg, lightly beaten

Directions

- Soak mushrooms in warm water for 30 minutes. Drain, cut off, and discard stems. Thinly slice caps.
- Bring broth to simmer, add chicken, and cook 3 minutes. Stir in vinegar, soy sauce, Tabasco, pepper, bamboo shoots, cilantro, green onion, and mushrooms. Return to simmer.
- Combine cornstarch and water. Stir into mixture. Simmer until slightly thickened, stirring constantly.
- Remove from heat and slowly drizzle in egg, stirring constantly.

Per Serving

calories 160

total fat 7g

saturated fat 2g

total carbohydrate 12g

dietary fiber less than 1g

protein 11g

Margaret Ferrazzi's Spiced Red Lentil Soup with Mint-Cilantro Raita

THIS EXOTIC LENTIL SOUP is rich in aroma but the hot Indian spices don't overwhelm. A dollop of the cooling yogurt relish will balance the flavors and add a creamy texture. Double your serving size and this vegan soup becomes a substantial main course. It'll keep for a week or more in the fridge.

Ingredients

6-8 servings

2 quarts of chicken broth, defatted
2 cups dry red lentils
3 large carrots
3 celery stalks
1 large brown onion, peeled
3 cloves garlic
2 inch chunk of ginger
¼ cup extra virgin olive oil
juice of ½ lime
salt and freshly ground black pepper to taste

Spice Mix:
1 tablespoon mild curry powder
1 tablespoon paprika
½ tablespoon turmeric
½ tablespoon garam masala
½ teaspoon ground cinnamon

Raita (Yogurt Relish):
1 pint nonfat plain yogurt
½ cup fresh cilantro leaves
½ cup fresh mint leaves
salt to taste

Directions

- Drain the yogurt by adding a little salt and putting it into a fine sieve set over a bowl. Place in the refrigerator. It's surprising how much water will be removed this way and it makes the nonfat yogurt nice and thick.

- Cut the carrots, celery, and onion in fine dice. Peel and mince the ginger and garlic finely. Combine the powdered spices until well mixed.
- Heat the olive oil in a large heavy saucepan. When very hot, add the diced vegetables. Stir briskly for a couple of minutes until they begin to release their juices and aromas. Add the garlic and ginger and stir, turn the heat to low and cover the pot tightly. Let these vegetables "sweat" for 10 minutes until softened.
- Stir in the spice mix and leave for a couple of minutes to let the dry spices cook to bring out the flavor. Add the chicken broth and the lentils and bring to a low boil. Cook uncovered until the lentils are tender (about 20 minutes). Do not overcook or they will become mushy.
- Add black pepper and salt to taste. The lime juice completes the seasoning.
- Chop the herbs fine and add to the yogurt. Pass the bowl of raita and help yourself.

Per Serving

calories 270
total fat 8g
saturated fat 1g

total carbohydrate 33g
dietary fiber 12g
protein 18g

Margaret Ferrazzi is a culinary consultant, cooking teacher, caterer, and chef to Hollywood celebrities and executives. Her clients have included Steven Spielberg, Ted Danson, Paul Reiser, and Matt Groening. Her love of aromatherapy and passion for fresh, seasonal foods is reflected in this recipe.

Michel Richard's Chicken, Mushroom, and Barley Soup

NOTHING COULD BE SIMPLER or more delicate than this dish. The flavors are rich and earthy. The texture creamy. It contains all the elements of a complete meal. It's nutritious and filling, to boot. I'm delighted that Michel Richard provided this recipe for *Diet Simple*. It fits perfectly as something you can cook, store in the refrigerator, and eat for several meals. And it's low in calories.

Ingredients

4 servings

- 2 tablespoons olive oil
- 2 small onions, peeled and diced
- 1 pound mushrooms, ends trimmed and thinly sliced
- 2 quarts unsalted chicken stock (defatted)
- ½ cup soy sauce
- 6 tablespoons pearl barley
- 4 cloves garlic, peeled and minced salt and freshly
- ground black pepper to taste
- 4 large chicken breasts or thighs, boned, skinned, and sliced into bite-size pieces, at room temperature
- 1½ cups (about 3 ounces) freshly grated Parmesan cheese (optional)

Directions

- Heat the oil in a heavy, medium-size saucepan over medium-low heat. Add the onion, cover, and cook until translucent, for about 10 minutes, stirring occasionally.
- Add the mushrooms, increase heat to medium-high, and cook uncovered until lightly browned, for about 5 minutes, stirring occasionally.

- Add the chicken stock, soy sauce, barley, and garlic. Simmer gently for 45 minutes to cook barley and then blend flavors.
- Season with salt and pepper.
- This can be prepared ahead, cooled, covered, and set aside at cool room temperature for up to 4 hours or refrigerated for several days.
- To serve, bring the soup to a boil, add chicken, reduce heat, and simmer just until the chicken becomes opaque, for about 2–3 minutes.
- Ladle into 4 soup plates. Pass Parmesan, if desired.

Per Serving Without Parmesan:
calories 320
total fat 10g
saturated fat 2g
total carbohydrate 26g
dietary fiber 6g
protein 34g

Per Serving With Parmesan:
calories 500
total fat 22g
saturated fat 9g
total carbohydrate 28g
dietary fiber 6g
protein 48g

Michel Richard and his latest restaurant, Citronelle, in Washington, D.C., have received numerous awards. In 2001, Zagat Survey named Citronelle one of the five best restaurants in Washington, D.C., and Gourmet magazine rated Citronelle in the top 20 of all restaurants in the United States. In 1988 Richard was inducted into the James Beard Foundation's "Who's Who in American Food and Wine." Richard is renowned as a genius with ingredients, using surprising combinations of textures and flavors.

Oodles Noodles' Spicy Chicken Noodle Soup

I LOVE TO STROLL down the street to Oodles Noodles, a local "noodle bar" in downtown Washington, D.C., and order this soup. The flavors explode in your mouth, and the combination of hot chili, lemongrass, Thai spices, and the fresh vegetables, noodles, and chicken makes this a full-course meal that's hard to beat.

If you want to make extra servings to save in your refrigerator, go ahead and cook the noodles and clean and chop the garnishes, but keep them in separate containers apart from the soup. The noodles are so delicate, they'll disintegrate if left in water. And it's nice to have crispy, fresh onions, bean sprouts, and cilantro to add at the last minute for maximum effect.

Ingredients

4 servings

½ pound bag Oriental style rice noodles (banh pho)
1 pound chicken breast
½ pound mushroom
4 stalks lemongrass stem
5 slices galangal
4 pieces kaffir lime leaves
7 cups chicken stock (defatted)
4–5 tablespoons fish sauce

4–5 tablespoons fresh lime juice
3–4 tablespoons Thai chili paste (namprik pao)

Garnish:
3 ounces spring onion (chopped)
3 ounces cilantro (chopped)
½ pound bean sprouts

(Note: the galangal and lime leaves are not edible. They're meant only to float in the bowl to impart their distinctive flavors.)

Directions

- Soak the rice noodles in cold water for at least 4 hours. Cut the chicken breast into thin slices. Slice the mushrooms. Set aside. Cut the lemongrass into short lengths.
- Add the lemongrass, galangal, and kaffir lime leaves to the chicken stock and bring to boil. Season to taste with fish sauce, lime juice, and chili paste, then bring to another boil. Add chicken and simmer until cooked, in a few minutes.
- Boil the noodles in hot water until soft, no more than 10 seconds.
- To serve, divide the noodles in 4, place in 4 soup bowls.
- Sprinkle on top of the noodles in each bowl one quarter of the bean sprouts, spring onions, and cilantro.
- Pour the hot soup over the noodles and garnish. Serve.

Chef's Note: Many of the ingredients, particularly the lemongrass, galangal, kaffir lime leaves, fish sauce and the oriental noodles, Banh Pho, can be found in an oriental market.

Per Serving

calories 460	total carbohydrate 62g
total fat 3.5	dietary fiber 6g
saturated fat 1g	protein 43g

Jessie Yan, *Vanessa Lim,* and **William Tu** *own Spices, Oodles Noodles, and Yanyu restaurants in Washington, D.C., all of which are popular and critically acclaimed. Oodles Noodles, an informal "noodle bar," has received rave reviews for serving fresh, light, innovative ingredients at very reasonable prices.*

Kjerstin's Crab Cakes

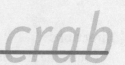

MY MOTHER'S recipe for crab cakes is very light, but tastes rich. These crab cakes are versatile, too. I've served them for brunch alongside fried eggs and hash browns and they make a great crabcake sandwich when placed between slices of toast.

You can hold the crabcake mixture in the refrigerator for up to three days and make fresh crabcakes in an instant.

4 servings

Ingredients

1 pound crab meat, fresh or canned
¼ cup breadcrumbs
1 egg
2 tablespoons reduced fat mayonnaise
1 tablespoon bay seasoning

½ tablespoon mustard
juice of 1 lemon
dash of Worchestershire sauce
dash of cayenne pepper
a few drops of Louisiana-style hot sauce (or Tabasco)

Directions

- Mix the crab meat lightly with the breadcrumbs. In a separate bowl, mix the egg, mayonnaise, bay seasoning, mustard, lemon juice, Worchestershire, cayenne pepper and hot sauce.
- Mix it all together and make 8 small patties.
- Fry in a pan over low to medium heat with a little oil, butter, or oil spray until lightly brown on each side.

Per Serving

calories 230
total fat 10g
saturated fat 1.5g

carbohydrate 7g
dietary fiber 0g
protein 26g

Patrick O'Connell's Chilled Charcoal Grilled Salmon in a Mustard Crust

THIS IS A DELIGHTFULLY different treatment for a whole salmon. The fish can be grilled ahead over charcoal and beautifully presented as a whole side, or it can be individually portioned and served chilled as a refreshing summery dish. The cooked salmon makes a versatile leftover flaked into a pasta salad, scrambled eggs, or a cocktail spread. Ask your fish supplier to split a whole salmon, removing the head and all of the bones, but leaving the skin, which helps keep the salmon intact on the grill. The salmon can be cooked under the broiler, as well.

9 servings

Ingredients

1 side of salmon, head and bones removed (about 3½ pounds with the skin on)

1 cup dried mustard seeds

1 bunch fresh dill, lightly chopped

1 medium onion, thinly sliced

¼ cup extra virgin olive oil

salt and freshly ground pepper to taste

For grilling: ½ pound hickory wood chips, optional

Directions

■ Lay the side of salmon flesh side up, salt and pepper liberally, and coat with the mustard seeds, then cover with the chopped dill, followed by thinly sliced raw onions. Finish with a sprinkling of olive oil.

■ Remove the rack from your charcoal grill and ignite the charcoal. Sprinkle the wood chips on top of the fire, letting the flames subside to glowing embers.

- Lay your rack on the top of the flesh side of the fish. Pressing the onions, dill, and seasonings in place with the rack, quickly flip the rack over the fire with the skin side facing up. Lower the lid if your grill has one and cook for 10 minutes. The fish will continue to cook somewhat after it is removed from the fire.

- To remove the fish from the fire use tongs or oven mitts to lift off the grill rack with the fish in place and set on a large metal tray or cookie sheet to cool. Gently remove the skin.

- To serve, place a serving tray or platter on top of the fish and holding the rack in place, turn the fish over onto the tray. Pick off and discard any burned bits of onion and dill.

- The salmon may be served whole or individually portioned by cutting into vertical strips approximately two inches wide.

Per Serving

calories 480

total fat 31g

saturated fat 5g

total carbohydrate 9g

dietary fiber 3g

protein 40g

Patrick O'Connell, chef and owner of the award-winning Inn at Little Washington, is a self-taught chef who pioneered a refined, regional American cuisine in the Virginia countryside. He has been referred to as "the Pope of American Haute Cuisine." America's first 5-star country house hotel, the Inn has been named "Restaurant of the Year" by the James Beard Foundation. O'Connell himself was named "Best Chef in the Mid-Atlantic region" and was recently honored with the "Outstanding Chef Award for 2001."

"Chilled Charcoal Grilled Salmon in a Mustard Seed Crust" is from **The Inn at Little Washington, A Consuming Passion**, published by Random House, 1996.

Dan Puzo's Red Wine Vinaigrette

DAN IS THE MASTER of salad dressings. I can't stop eating his salads. This vinaigrette is rich, with just the right amount of tartness.

I use it on a simple tossed green salad, cucumbers and tomatoes, or as a marinade for chilled asparagus. Toss it into sliced leftover steak with some chopped vegetables.

Ingredients

12 servings

½ cup red wine vinegar
⅓ cup red wine, such as California Cabernet Sauvignon
½ cup extra virgin olive oil
1 tablespoon dried basil or ⅛ cup fresh basil

1 teaspoon dried oregano or 2 tablespoons fresh oregano
1 teaspoon sea salt
½ teaspoon garlic powder, optional
dash black pepper, optional

Directions

- In deep bowl, mix red wine vinegar, red wine, olive oil, basil, oregano, and salt. Add garlic powder and/or black pepper, if desired.
- Whisk until blended. Makes about 1½ cups.

Per 2-Tablespoon Serving

calories 90
total fat 9g
saturated fat 1.5g

total carbohydrate 2g
dietary fiber 0g
protein 0g

Dan Puzo *is an 18-year veteran of the* Los Angeles Times, *where he won two James Beard Awards for food journalism. He is also a wine columnist with a passion for California wines.*

East Coast Grill and Raw Bar's Chickpea Salad with Cumin and Mint

I LOVE A SPICY, hearty salad with a lot of different elements—crunch, tartness, sweetness, and heat. And they're all in this dish. And so are all the nutritional elements that make this a perfect one-pot meal. I bring this dish to a spring or summer pot luck and people are thrilled with the flavors. I love serving it as a main course for a simple lunch. It's a versatile recipe and can be stored in the refrigerator for a week for many meals for you and your family. Double or triple it so you'll have plenty!

4 servings

Ingredients

1 cup dried chickpeas or 1 15-ounce can chickpeas

1 tablespoon salt (if using dried chickpeas)

⅓ cup olive oil

¼ cup fresh lemon juice (about 1 lemon)

1 tablespoon minced garlic

1 red bell pepper, halved, seeded, and diced medium

½ cup roughly chopped scallions (white and green parts)

¼ cup roughly chopped fresh mint

2 tablespoon cumin seeds, toasted if you want, or 1 tablespoon ground cumin

1 tablespoon minced jalapeno or other fresh chili pepper of your choice (optional)

2 bunches watercress, trimmed, washed, and dried

Directions

■ If you are using dried chickpeas place them in a large pot, cover with water, and let soak overnight, or for at least 5 hours. Drain and rinse 2 or 3 times.

- Return the chickpeas to the pot, cover with water again, add salt, and bring to a boil over high heat. Immediately reduce the heat to medium and simmer for 1 hour to 1 hour and 15 minutes, or until the chickpeas are tender but not mushy. Drain and rinse thoroughly with cold water. If you are using canned chickpeas, simply drain and rinse them.
- Place the chickpeas in a medium bowl, add all the remaining ingredients except the watercress, and toss well. Cover and refrigerate until well chilled, at least 30 minutes. When chilled, place the watercress on a platter or individual serving plates, top with the chickpea salad, and serve.

Per Serving

calories 370	total carbohydrate 36g
total fat 21g	dietary fiber 10g
saturated fat 3g	protein 11g

Chris Schlesinger is the chef and co-owner of the East Coast Grill, named one of Boston's "Top 20 Restaurants" in the Zagat Survey 2001. **John Wiloughby** is senior editor of Cook's Illustrated. Schlesinger and Wiloughby are authors of Lettuce in Your Kitchen, Big Flavors of the Hot Sun, and License to Grill, among other books.

"Chickpea Salad with Cumin and Mint" is excerpted from License to Grill, published by William Morrow and Company, Inc., 1997.

Gerard Pangaud's Salad of Cod with Citrus

THIS IS AN ELEGANT dish from one of the top French chefs in the country. It is a wonderful first course, but I prefer to double the recipe and the serving size for weeklong main courses. The citrus fruit is a perfect accompaniment with the fish. It doesn't overpower, only complements and adds depth. You'll be transported to an island in the Mediterranean with just one bite.

4 servings

Ingredients

1 10- to 12-ounce cod filet, with skin
½ teaspoon ground dried ginger
½ teaspoon ground dried coriander
¼ teaspoon dried nutmeg
½ teaspoon anis seed

1 pinch ground clove
¼ teaspoon ground cumin
1 orange, plus zest
1 lemon, plus zest
1 lime, plus zest
¼ grapefruit
⅓ cup olive oil
¼ pound arugula

Directions

- Preheat the oven to 375 degrees and mix all the spices.
- Using about ⅔ of the olive oil, brush the fish and coat the baking dish. Reserve ⅓ of the oil for use later. Place the fish in the baking dish skin side down. Spread the spices on top of the fish and put in the oven for approximately 8–12 minutes depending on the thickness of the fish.
- Grate the skin of the orange, lemon, and lime being careful to use only the colorful zest, not the white part of the

skin. Peel the orange, lemon, lime, and grapefruit and separate the fruits into sections.

■ Take the fish out of the oven and flake it. Deglaze the baking dish by adding the rest of the olive oil and pulling up the bits of fish left in the bottom of the pan. Put the flavored oil in a bowl and add the citrus sections, tossing well.

■ Place the cod harmoniously with the arugula on a plate and spoon the citrus relish over the fish.

■ Serve warm.

Per Serving

calories 260	total carbohydrate 10g
total fat 19g	dietary fiber 3g
saturated fat 2.5g	protein 14g

Gerard Pangaud opened Gerard's Place in downtown Washington, D.C., in 1993 and has been lauded by the critics ever since. For the past 4 years he has been awarded 4 Stars in the Mobil Guide as well as by Washingtonian magazine. The Zagat Survey consistently lists Gerard's Place in the top 5 restaurants in Washington, D.C.

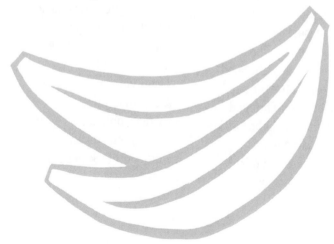

Najmieh Batmanglij's Persian Chicken Salad

THIS IS A BEAUTIFUL CHICKEN salad, with a perfect harmony of flavors, colors, and textures. I love to serve it for a ladies lunch or a summer picnic. My friends and clients who have sampled it are delighted with the unique combination of vegetables, chicken, herbs, and spices. It's a filling comfort food with the added lightness of fresh vegetables and the tang of a great dressing. I call it Nouvelle Persian!

12 servings

Ingredients

1 frying chicken, about 2 or 3 pounds, with skin removed

1 onion, peeled and finely chopped

1 teaspoon salt

4 carrots, peeled and chopped

2 cups fresh shelled or frozen green peas

2 scallions, chopped

2 celery stalks, chopped

5 large potatoes, boiled, peeled, and chopped

3 medium cucumber pickles, finely chopped (dill pickles—polish or kosher are best)

½ cup chopped fresh parsley

⅔ cup green olives, pitted and chopped

3 hard-boiled eggs, peeled and chopped (optional)

Dressing

1 cup defatted chicken broth

3 cups light mayonnaise

2 tablespoons dijon mustard

¼ cup olive oil

¼ cup vinegar

¼ cup lime juice

1½ teaspoon salt

½ teaspoon freshly ground black pepper

Directions

- Place the chicken in a nonstick pot along with the onion and salt. Cover and cook for 1½ hours over low heat (no water is added because chicken makes its own juice). When done, allow to cool, debone the chicken, and chop finely. Set aside the chicken broth for later use.
- Steam the carrots for 5 minutes and set aside.
- Steam shelled peas for 5 minutes and set aside. (If using frozen peas, follow package directions.)
- In a large bowl, whisk together chicken broth, mayonnaise, mustard, olive oil, vinegar, lime juice, salt and pepper. Mix thoroughly.
- Combine chicken, prepared vegetables and eggs with the rest of the ingredients. Pour the dressing over it and toss well. Adjust seasoning to taste.
- Chill for at least 2 hours.

Per Serving

calories 480	total carbohydrate 29g
total fat 29g	dietary fiber 4g
saturated fat 5g	protein 26g

Persian Chicken Salad is from Persian Cooking for a Healthy Kitchen, *by **Najmieh Batmanglij**. Persian cooking is unique in its imaginative use of spices. This book combines the best of Persian cuisine with healthy living.*

© *1994–2001 courtesy of Mage Publishers, Washington, D.C.*

Phyllis Frucht's Black Bean and Mango Salad with Citrus Herb Dressing

THIS IS A SPICY AND LIGHT SALAD with all the elements of a great main course—hearty beans, sweet mango, crunchy pepper and onion, tart lime juice, hot jalapeno. This dish is quick to prepare and perfect for an individual summer dinner. Double or triple the recipe so you'll have plenty for the week.

6 servings

Ingredients

2 cans black beans, drained and rinsed

2 mangos, peeled and diced

2 red bell peppers, seeded and diced

1 cup red onion, diced

½ cup lime juice

½ cup orange juice

2 tablespoons honey

2 tablespoons lime zest

2 tablespoons orange zest

2 tablespoons Herbes de Provence

2 jalapeno peppers, seeded and minced

½ cup cilantro, chopped

Directions

- Combine the beans, mango, red pepper, and onion in a bowl. Mix the rest of the ingredients. Toss well and serve.

Per Serving

calories 220

total fat 2g

saturated fat 0g

total carbohydrate 46g

dietary fiber 10g

protein 10g

Phyllis Frucht is a chef and teacher in Washington, D.C., specializing in international cuisine from the Orient to India, Europe, the Middle East, the Caribbean, and more.

Roberto Donna's White Bean and Shrimp Salad with Basil Dressing

I HAVE MADE THIS RECIPE so many times I can't keep track. I've not met one person who can resist the flavorful combination of cold beans and shrimp lathered in basil and balsamic vinegar. I take it to picnics, pot lucks, and use it as a main course for lunch or dinner. It's a delightfully light and flavorful summer meal that won't tire your taste buds for a week.

Ingredients

4 servings

8 ounces dry cannellini beans (or 24 oz canned, rinsed)

½ peeled onion

1 celery stalk

4 sage leaves

½ medium carrot

8 ounces shrimp

2 cups white wine

2 tablespoons balsamic vinegar

6 tablespoons extra virgin olive oil

10 basil leaves

salt and pepper to taste

Directions

- Soak the cannellini beans in water for 12 hours; drain, and place in a pot of water, add salt and pepper; cover and simmer for 45 minutes.
- Chop and add the onion, celery, and carrot, cooking another 10 minutes. Add the finely diced sage to the pot and drain the cooking liquid. Place in a cool location.
- Wash and clean the shrimp and poach for 3 minutes, or until done, in the white wine.
- Add salt and pepper to taste.

main dish salads

- Dressing: Finely chop basil and add the balsamic vinegar, salt, pepper, and olive oil. Whisk until emulsified.
- Place ¼ of the mixture on each plate and top with 2 ounces of the shrimp. Dress with the basil dressing.

Per Serving

calories 540	total carbohydrate 41g
total fat 23g	dietary fiber 15g
saturated fat 3.5g	protein 24g

As a James Beard Award-winning chef and restaurateur in Washington, D.C., **Roberto Donna** *is committed to introducing others to the real flavors of Italy. In 1984 he opened Galileo and gained a strong following, and in 1997,* Wine Spectator *called Galileo one of the "10 Best Italian Restaurants in America." The magazine has presented Mr. Donna with the "Grand Award of Excellence" every year since 1997. Galileo was also named one of the twenty finest Italian restaurants in the world by the president of Italy.*

284 ■ main dish salads

> The *Diet Simple* strategies alone will work. But if you'd like to take a more scientific approach to weight loss, these next two sections are for you.

Appendix

The Metabolism Toolbox

A growing body of scientific evidence confirms that the human body is an extraordinarily adaptive and delicate instrument whose instinctive drive for survival complicates the plans of even the most dedicated dieter. Losing weight and keeping it off require a careful understanding of the body and, specifically, its metabolic needs.

The less you eat, the more your body's metabolism slows down, requiring you to eat even less. And when, out of frustration or exhaustion, you resume "normal" eating, your body grabs onto those extra calories and sends them into fat storage with a vengeance.

Your body's calorie needs are largely determined by two factors: your level of physical activity and your resting metabolic rate (RMR).

About one-third of the calories you burn are the result of physical activity, which includes anything other than resting—brushing your teeth, folding clothes, working at your computer, walking around the block, or exercising in your health club.

The other two-thirds are the calories needed to sustain basic bodily functioning: maintaining body temperature, heart beat, breathing, organ repair, and basic chemical reactions. This is your resting metabolic rate. Because RMR accounts for a large majority of calories burned, keeping your RMR high is essential to losing weight and keeping it off.

All of which raises the questions: How do you find out what your RMR is? And how can you raise it?

Your RMR is influenced by a variety of factors including genetics, body size, muscle mass, age, gender, body weight, pregnancy, hormonal status and, yes, physical condition. (A fit and muscular body burns more calories while at rest than an unfit, less muscular one.) To make things more difficult, RMR naturally declines through adulthood at about 2 percent per decade, usually because of the muscle loss you experience as you age and become more sedentary. Chronic dieters exacerbate muscle loss through repeated quick weight reductions.

You can determine your estimated resting metabolic rate (RMR) using *Diet Simple*'s formula. Then continue the calculation to account for your level of physical activity and see how many calories you need to eat just to maintain your weight. Next, subtract 250 to 500 calories to determine your best daily calorie level for producing a ½ to 1 pound per week weight loss. But your calorie intake should never go below your RMR and ideally, even for the lower calorie levels, should always be at least 150 calories above.

Once you've done the math, spend at least one week—or up to a month—eating at that calorie level, to see if you are losing weight at the desired pace. If you do not lose weight, and you're sure you've calculated your calorie needs and your food intake correctly (cheating here will do you no good, folks), then that's the sign your metabolism is probably low.

A low metabolism makes it almost impossible to lose weight or even maintain a weight loss. If you think you're low, you may benefit from visiting a doctor and getting tested to verify your metabolic status or if your thyroid is functioning properly.

If everything checks out, and your doctor determines you don't need a medication, eating a healthy diet, exercising, and muscle building are the only ways a low metabolism can be reversed safely and effectively.

Three factors, then, are necessary in order to lose weight.

First, raise your metabolism level with a muscle-building program. The more lean muscle you have, the more calories your body burns. The American College of Sports Medicine recommends strength training all of your major muscle groups twice a week.

Second, cardiovascular activity burns body fat and calories (and, of course, improves your heart and general health). A fit body also continues to burn more calories even after the workout has ended. Accumulate at least 30 minutes per day of cardiovascular activity for health and weight maintenance. You may need to exercise more to lose weight.

The third element is diet. If you want to lose weight without affecting your metabolism negatively, the key is keeping calories as high as possible—but still slightly lower than what is needed to maintain weight. The metabolic experts recommend a daily caloric deficit of no more than 250 to 500 calories below the calorie level necessary to maintain your weight. Using the formula that 3,500 calories equals one pound, a daily deficit of 250 to 500 calories would produce losses of ½ to 1 pound every week.

Diet Simple's Formula* for Calculating Your Resting Metabolic Rate and Calorie Needs

* Based on the Harris Benedict Equation for people over 17 years old

WOMEN		
1. Begin with a base of 655 calories		655
2. Multiply your weight in pounds by 4.3		
3. Multiply your height in inches by 4.7		
4. Add together the totals from #1, #2, and #3		
5. Multiply your age by 4.7		
6. Subtract result of #5 from total of #4 (*your normal Resting Metabolic Rate*)		
7. Multiply #6 by your activity factor (*your daily maintenance calories*)		
8. Subtract 250–500 calories (*your daily weight loss calories*)		

FOR ACTIVITY, MULTIPLY:

RMR times 1.2 for low levels of activity (sedentary)

RMR times 1.3 for light exercise (about 2–3 hours per week)

RMR times 1.4 for moderate physical activity (about 4–7 hours per week), and

RMR times 1.6 for high levels of activity (about 7+ hours per week: high levels of exercise or manual labor)

Some athletes may double or even triple their RMR to determine their daily calorie needs

MEN		
1.	Begin with a base of 66 calories	66
2.	Multiply your weight in pounds by 6.3	
3.	Multiply your height in inches by 12.7	
4.	Add together the totals from #1, #2, and #3	
5.	Multiply your age by 6.8	
6.	Subtract result of #5 from total of #4 (*your normal Resting Metabolic Rate*)	
7.	Multiply #6 by your activity factor (*your daily maintenance calories*)	
8.	Subtract 250–500 calories (*your daily weight loss calories*)	

FOR ACTIVITY, MULTIPLY:

RMR times 1.2 for low levels of activity (sedentary)

RMR times 1.3 for light exercise (about 2–3 hours per week)

RMR times 1.4 for moderate physical activity (about 4–7 hours per week), and

RMR times 1.6 for high levels of activity (about 7+ hours per week: high levels of exercise or manual labor)

Some athletes may double or even triple their RMR to determine their daily calorie needs

EXAMPLES

1. 150-pound, 5'4" 40-year-old moderately exercising woman:	
1. Begin with a base of 655 calories	655
2. Multiply your weight in pounds by 4.3	645
3. Multiply your height in inches by 4.7	301
4. Add together the totals from #1, #2, and #3	TOTAL = 1,601
5. Multiply your age by 4.7	subtract: -188
6. Subtract result of #5 from total of #4 (*your normal Resting Metabolic Rate*)	RMR = 1,413
7. Calories to maintain weight (RMR x 1.4)	1,978 calories per day
8. Calories to lose weight (subtract 250–500)	1,498–1,728 calories per day

2. 200-pound, 6'1" 50-year-old highly active man:	
1. Begin with a base of 66 calories	66
2. Multiply your weight in pounds by 6.3	1,260
3. Multiply your height in inches by 12.7	+927
4. Add together the totals from #1, #2, and #3	TOTAL = 2,253
5. Multiply your age by 6.8	subtract: -340
6. Subtract result of #5 from total of #4 (*your normal Resting Metabolic Rate*)	RMR = 1,913
7. Calories to maintain weight (RMR x 1.6)	3,060 calories per day
8. Calories to lose weight (subtract 500)	2,560 calories per day

Appendix
Diet Simple Menu Plans

I've designed these menus to be delicious tasting, simple and quick to prepare, and perfectly balanced so you will feel completely satisfied with each meal even though you're eating fewer calories than your body needs—for weight loss.

Your health and satisfaction with your meals depends on eating a wide variety of foods each day. The following meals are perfectly balanced among all of the elements:

Fruits and Vegetables

Probably the most important part of your meals is the fruits and vegetables. Of course, you already know that. That's why *Diet Simple* is so full of practical tips for how you can eat more and make them delicious additions to your meals. Think of each fruit and vegetable as a little factory of nutrients and beneficial substances—called phytochemicals—with potent powers of healing and disease prevention.

For weight loss, fruits and vegetables are critical as they add fiber, bulk, and quantity to your meals to help you feel nice and full.

Whole Grains

Most of *Diet Simple*'s meals contain a whole grain, which provides fiber and satisfaction. Studies show people who eat more fiber, especially at breakfast, feel less hungry the whole day, and that means it's easier to lose weight. The nutrients in a whole grain are correlated with a decrease in many types of cancer, heart disease, and even diabetes. But 75 percent of a grain's nutritional value is removed when it is refined to make white flour. So it's worth it to make the switch—especially considering the superior flavor and texture you'll get from the whole grain.

Protein

Diet Simple's menus are chock full of protein, either as hearty beans, lean red meat, poultry, or seafood. I stress fish as the most ideal protein source because of the presence of important omega-3 fatty acids—and the wonderful flavor. Research shows omega-3s may prevent a host of health problems such as depression, inflammatory diseases, and high cholesterol.

Fat

Recent studies confirm that people who lose weight and keep it off successfully eat a low-fat diet. And since I can't argue with success, that's what I recommend. But you do have to eat fat at every meal. You need it to feel full and to make your food taste good. You will find most of *Diet Simple*'s menus contain about 20–30 percent fat calories, which is the ideal recommended by all the experts. You also may notice that the majority of fat used in the menus is monounsaturated or polyunsaturated, which are more beneficial for your health. Saturated fat and trans fat are definitely hard to find in these menus. I recommend them only for an occasional indulgence!

Which Menus Should I Follow?

To determine which set of menus will work best for you, calculate your calorie needs, then divide by 3 and distribute equally among breakfast, lunch, and dinner.

If your calorie needs are 1,500, give yourself a 500-calorie breakfast, a 500-calorie lunch, and a 500-calorie dinner. If you need 2,400 calories per day, the 800-calorie meals would be best for you. For the lower calorie levels, I recommend eating a minimum 500-calorie breakfast, with smaller meals later. So, for instance, if you want to eat 1,300 calories per day, eat a 500-calorie breakfast, a 400-calorie lunch, and a 400-calorie dinner. I've even provided examples of dinners as low as 300 calories. This will enable you to eat adequate breakfasts and lunches, a snack or two in between, and a light dinner.

I have found that people do their best, crave less, overeat less, and feel most in control when they eat adequate calories during the day. This also enables you not to attack dinner and to eat lighter at night, a very successful strategy for weight loss.

400-CALORIE BALANCED BREAKFASTS
Simple Breakfast
cold cereal (150), 1 cup skim milk (100)
½ oz (⅛ cup) nuts (80)
4 oz fresh fruit or juice (60)

Katherine's Favorite Breakfast
½ cup old-fashioned oats (150), cooked in:
1 cup skim milk (100) or soy milk
pinch salt
2 whole chopped walnuts (50)
Microwave 5 minutes in a large bowl (to prevent it from
    spilling over), leave in microwave another minute

Stir in:
1 tsp brown sugar (15)
On the side: ½ cup orange juice (60)

Peanut Butter "To Go" Breakfast
2 slices whole grain bread (160)
1 tbsp peanut butter (90)
6–8 oz fat-free yogurt (90)
4 oz fresh-fruit or juice (60)

Egg and Sausage Breakfast
¼ cup egg substitute (50)
1 tbsp olive oil (120)
Or
2 eggs (150) and 1 tsp oil (40)
Scramble in:
½ cup chopped onion and garlic (20)
1 oz lean sausage or ham (50)
½ whole wheat English muffin or 1 slice whole wheat toast (80)
½ cup orange juice (60)

Lox and Bagel "To Go" Breakfast
2 oz whole wheat bagel (160)
4 oz lox (140)
1 tbsp fat-free cream cheese (30)
4 oz juice (60)

400-CALORIE SIMPLE, BALANCED LUNCHES OR DINNERS
4 oz halibut or white fish (105)
1 tsp olive oil, herbs, salt (40)

sautéed or steamed vegetables (50)
1–6 oz baked potato (160)
Top with:
2 tbsp fat-free sour cream topping or ¼ cup 1% cottage
   cheese (30)

½ cup cooked (1 oz raw) whole wheat pasta (100)
4 oz chicken breast or tuna (140)
Stirred into:
½ cup stir-fried diced tomatoes, capers (50)
2 tbsp grated Parmesan cheese (50)
1 piece fruit (60)

Stir-Fried Shrimp (or Chicken or Tofu) and Vegetables
1 cup cooked (or 2 oz raw) brown rice (200)
4 oz shrimp or chicken breast or ¾ cup tofu (140)
1–2 cups raw vegetables (50)
Stir-fried in 1 tsp sesame oil (40)

4 oz grilled chicken breast (140)
1 slice (1 oz) whole grain roll (80)
sautéed, sliced red and yellow peppers (25)
1 tbsp oil (120)
1 piece fruit (60)

3 oz grilled salmon (150)
6 oz boiled new potatoes with skin (boiled 15 minutes, check
   for doneness) (160)
1 tsp olive oil with parsley drizzled over potatoes (40)
1 cup fresh greens salad (25)
low-calorie salad dressing (25)

1 small whole wheat tortilla (130)
Filled with:
4 oz refried beans or canned, rinsed black beans (100)
1 oz cheese (100)
¾ cup salsa (75)

1 cup brown rice and beans (200)
1 oz baked chips for dipping (100)
½ cup fresh salsa (50)
⅙ of an avocado (50)

Simple Good Old American "To Go" Lunch
Sandwich: 2 slices bread (160), ½ tbsp mayo (50), 3 oz lean
    beef, turkey, seafood, or chicken breast (150)
Vegetable salad (25–50), 2 tbsp fat-free salad dressing (20)

500-CALORIE BALANCED BREAKFASTS
Simple Breakfast
cold cereal (200), 1 cup skim milk (100)
½ oz (⅛ cup) nuts (80)
8 oz fresh fruit and/or juice (120)

Katherine's Favorite Breakfast
½ cup old-fashioned oats (150), cooked in:
1 cup skim milk (100) or soy milk
pinch salt
2 whole chopped walnuts (50) (¼ cup walnuts, about 1 oz =
    200 calories)
Microwave 5 minutes in a large bowl (it will spill over), leave
    in microwave another minute
Add:
1 tsp brown sugar (15)

1 tbsp light butter (50)
½ medium banana or ½ cup blueberries (50)
On the side: ½ cup orange juice (60)

Peanut Butter "To Go" Breakfast
2 slices whole grain bread (160)
2 tbsp peanut butter (180)
6–8 oz fat-free yogurt (90), 4 oz fruit/juice (60)

Egg and Sausage Breakfast
¼ cup egg substitute (50)
1 tbsp olive oil (120)
Or
2 eggs (150) and 1 tsp oil (40)
Scramble in:
½ cup chopped onion and garlic (20)
1 oz lean sausage or ham (50)
whole wheat English muffin or 2 slices toast (160)
4 oz fresh fruit or juice (60)

Lox and Bagel "To Go" Breakfast
2½ oz whole wheat bagel (200)—that would be half of a large
    5 oz bagel (bagels are 80 cal/oz)
4 oz lox (140)
1 oz cream cheese (100)
4 oz juice (60)

500-CALORIE SIMPLE, BALANCED LUNCHES OR DINNERS
4 oz halibut or white fish (140)
1 tsp olive oil, herbs, salt (40)
sautéed or steamed vegetables (50)
1–6 oz baked potato (160)

Top with:
2 tbsp sour cream or ½ cup 2% cottage cheese (100)

1 cup cooked (2 oz raw) whole wheat pasta (200)
4 oz chicken breast or tuna (140)
Stirred in:
½ cup stir-fried diced tomatoes, capers (50)
2 tbsp grated Parmesan cheese (50)
1 piece fruit (60)

Stir-Fried Shrimp (or Chicken or Tofu) and Vegetables
1 cup brown rice (200)
4 oz shrimp or chicken breast or ¾ cup tofu (140)
1–2 cups raw vegetables (50)
Stir-fried in 1 tbsp sesame oil (120)

4 oz grilled chicken breast (140)
2 slices (ounces) whole grain roll (160)
sautéed, sliced red and yellow peppers (25)
1 tbsp oil or 2 tbsp regular salad dressing (120)
1 piece fruit (60)

4 oz grilled salmon (200)
6 oz boiled new potatoes (boiled 15 minutes, check for
    doneness) (160)
1 tsp olive oil with parsley drizzled over potatoes (40)
1 cup salad greens or grated cabbage (25)
2 tbsp reduced-calorie salad dressing (50)

1 small whole wheat tortilla (130)
Filled with:

4 oz refried beans or canned, rinsed black beans (100)
1 oz cheese (100)
½ cup salsa (50)
½ avocado (150)

1½ cups beans and rice (300)
Sautéed in 1 tbsp oil (120)
½ cup salsa (50)

Simple Good Old American "To Go" Lunch
Sandwich: 2 slices bread (160), 1 tbsp mayo (100), 3 oz lean
    beef, turkey, seafood, or chicken breast (150)
Vegetable salad (25–50), 2 tbsp low-calorie salad dressing
    (75)

600-CALORIE BALANCED BREAKFASTS
Easy Breakfast
cold cereal (280), 1 cup skim milk (100)
½ oz or about ⅛ cup chopped walnuts (80)
8 oz fresh fruit and/or juice (120)

Katherine's Favorite Breakfast
½ cup old-fashioned oats (150) or cold cereal
1 cup skim milk (100) or soy milk
pinch salt
1 oz (¼ cup) chopped nuts (160)
Microwave 5 minutes in a large bowl (to prevent it from
    spilling over), leave in microwave another minute
Mix in:
1 tsp brown sugar (20)
1 tbsp light butter (50)

Top with:
½ sliced medium banana, ½ cup blueberries or other fresh fruit (50)
½ cup juice (60)

Peanut Butter "To Go" Breakfast
2 slices whole grain bread (160)
2 tbsp peanut butter (180)
8 oz yogurt (200)
4 oz fresh fruit or juice (60)

Eggs and Sausage Breakfast
½ cup egg substitute (100)
1 tbsp olive oil (120)
Or
2 eggs (150) and 1 tsp oil (40)
Scramble in:
½ cup chopped onion and garlic (50)
whole wheat English muffin or 2 slices whole wheat toast (160)
½ cup orange juice (60)
½ large banana or other fruit (60)

Lox and Bagel "To Go" Breakfast
4 oz whole wheat bagel (300) (bagels are about 80 calories per oz)
4 oz lox (140)
1 oz cream cheese (100)
4 oz juice or fresh fruit (60)

600-CALORIE SIMPLE, BALANCED DINNERS OR LUNCHES

6 oz halibut or white fish (210)
1 tbsp olive oil, herbs, salt (120)
1–2 cups raw, sautéed, or steamed vegetables (50)
1 6-oz baked potato (160)
Top with:
3 tbsp reduced-fat sour cream or ½ cup 1% cottage cheese (75)

1½ cups cooked (3 oz raw) whole wheat pasta (300)
4 oz chicken breast or tuna (140)
1 cup stir fried diced tomatoes, capers (50)
1 tbsp olive oil (120)

Stir-Fried Shrimp (or Chicken or Tofu) and Vegetables:
1½ cups brown rice (300)
4 oz shrimp or chicken breast or ¾ cup tofu (140)
1–2 cups raw vegetables (50)
Stir-fried in 1 tbsp sesame oil (120)

6 oz grilled chicken breast marinated in fat-free Italian dressing (210)
1 medium (6 oz) Yukon Gold or Idaho potato (160) shredded and cooked in ½ tbsp olive oil (60)
1–2 cups sliced red and yellow peppers, raw or sautéed (50)
1 tbsp oil (120)

4 oz grilled salmon (200)
1 4-inch acorn squash, baked (45 minutes, check for doneness) (170)
1 tbsp olive oil and parsley drizzled over potatoes (120)
1 cup salad greens and/or grated cabbage (25)
2 tbsp reduced-calorie salad dressing or 1 tbsp regular (75)

1½ cups beans/rice (300)
1 oz cheese (100)
1 cup salad greens and/or grated cabbage (25)
⅓ avocado (100)
2 tbsp reduced-calorie salad dressing or 1 tbsp regular (75)

Simple Good Old American "To Go" Lunch
Sandwich: 2 slices whole grain bread (160), 1 tbsp mayo
      (100), 3 oz lean beef or turkey or chicken breast (150)
Vegetable salad (25-50), 2 tbsp regular salad dressing (130)

FOR PEOPLE WHO EAT DINNER TOO LATE (AND DON'T WANT TO ATTACK IT)
600-calorie dinner divided into:
300-calorie afternoon or early evening snack plus 300-calorie
      dinner

300-CALORIE SIMPLE, QUICK, AND EASY SNACK IDEAS
Snack 1:
Fruit, crackers, or bread (100) with 2 tbsp peanut butter
      (180)
Snack 2:
Fruit (60) and yogurt (240)
Snack 3:
Fruit (140) and 1 oz (¼ cup) nuts (160)
Snack 4:
Frozen dinner (300)

300-CALORIE SIMPLE, BALANCED LUNCHES AND DINNERS
3 oz halibut or white fish (105)
2 tsp olive oil, herbs, salt (80)

1 cup raw, sautéed, or steamed vegetables (25)
1–3 oz potato (80)

½ cup cooked (1 oz dry) whole wheat pasta (100)
3 oz chicken breast or tuna (105)
Stirred into:
½ cup diced tomatoes, capers, or 50 calories' worth of tomato
    sauce (50)
2 tbsp grated Parmesan cheese (50)

Stir-Fried Shrimp (or Chicken or Tofu) and Vegetables
½ cups cooked (1 oz raw) brown rice (100)
3 oz shrimp or chicken breast or ½ cup tofu (105)
1–2 cups raw vegetables (50),
Sautéed in 1 tsp sesame oil (40)

3 oz grilled chicken breast (105)
1 slice (1 oz) whole grain roll (80)
1–2 cups sautéed, sliced red and yellow peppers or other veg-
    etables (50)
1 tsp oil (40)

3 oz grilled salmon (150)
1 cup green salad or grated cabbage (25)
2 tbsp regular salad dressing (130)

1 small whole wheat tortilla (130)
4 oz refried beans or canned, rinsed black beans (100)
½ cup salsa (50)

½ cup brown rice and beans (100)
½ cup fresh salsa (50)
1 oz baked chips (100) for dipping
2 tbsp reduced-fat sour cream (50)

700-CALORIE BALANCED BREAKFASTS

Easy Breakfast
Cereal (230), 1½ cups skim milk (150)
1 oz (¼ cup) nuts (180)
8 oz fresh fruit and/or juice (120)

Katherine's Favorite Breakfast
½ cup old-fashioned oats (150)
1 cup skim milk or soy milk (100)
pinch salt
1 oz (¼ cup) chopped walnuts (160)
Microwave 5 minutes in a large bowl (to prevent it from
    spilling over), leave in microwave another minute
Add:
2 tsp brown sugar (30)
2 tbsp light butter (100)
½ large banana or 1 cup blueberries or other fruit (60)
½ cup orange juice (60)

Egg and Sausage Breakfast
½ cup egg substitute (100)
1 tbsp olive oil (120)
Or
3 eggs (225) and 1 tsp olive oil (40)
Scramble in:
½ cup chopped onion and garlic (25)
3 oz lean sausage or ham (130)

whole wheat English muffin or 2 slices toast (160)
½ cup orange juice (60)
½ large banana or 4 oz other fresh fruit (60)

Peanut Butter "To Go" Breakfast
8 oz low-fat yogurt (210)
2 slices whole wheat toast (160)
2 tbsp peanut butter (200)
8 oz fresh fruit or juice (120)

Lox and Bagel "To Go" Breakfast
4 oz bagel (320)
4 oz lox (140)
1 oz cream cheese (100)
8 oz fruit and/or juice (120)

700-CALORIE DINNERS OR LUNCHES
6 oz halibut or white fish (210)
1 tbsp olive oil, herbs, salt (120)
1–2 cups raw, sautéed, or steamed vegetables (50)
1 9-oz baked potato (240)
2 tbsp reduced-fat sour cream (40)
3 oz wine or 4 oz fruit or juice (60)

1½ cups cooked (3 ounces dry) whole wheat pasta (300)
5 oz chicken breast or tuna (175)
1 cup stir fried diced tomatoes, capers (100)
1 tbsp olive oil (120)

Stir-Fried Shrimp (or Chicken or Tofu) and Vegetables
1½ cups (or 3 oz dry) brown rice (300)
6 oz shrimp or chicken breast or 1 cup tofu (210)

1–2 cups raw chopped vegetables (50)
Stir-fried in 1 tbsp sesame oil (120)

6 oz grilled salmon (300)
6 oz boiled new potatoes (boiled 15 minutes, check for doneness) (160)
1 tbsp olive oil and parsley drizzled over potatoes (120)
1 cup salad greens and/or grated cabbage (25)
2 tbsp reduced-calorie salad dressing (75)

4 oz sliced chicken breast (140)
2 cups red beans mixed with rice (400)
Sautéed vegetables in (25) ½ tbsp oil or 2 tbsp salad dressing (120)

Simple Good Old American "To Go" Lunch
Sandwich: 2 slices bread (160), 1 tbsp mayo (100), 6 oz lean beef or turkey or chicken breast (210)
Vegetable salad (25), 3 tbsp regular salad dressing (225)

800-CALORIE BALANCED BREAKFASTS
Simple Breakfast
cereal (400)
1 cup skim milk (100)
1 oz (¼ cup) nuts (160)
8 oz fresh fruit and/or juice (120)

Katherine's Favorite Breakfast
¾ cup old-fashioned oats (225) or cold cereal
1½ cup skim milk (150)
pinch salt
1 oz (¼ cup) chopped walnuts (160)

Microwave 5 minutes in large bowl (to prevent it from spilling over), leave in microwave another minute

Mix in:

1 tbsp brown sugar (45)

2 tbsp light butter (100)

Top with:

½ large banana or ¾ cup blueberries or other fruit (60)

½ cup orange juice (60)

Peanut Butter "To Go" Breakfast

3 slices whole wheat toast (240)

3 tbsp peanut butter (270)

8 oz fresh fruit and/or juice (120)

yogurt (170)

Egg and Sausage Breakfast

¾ cup egg substitute (75)

1½ tbsp olive oil (180)

Or

3 eggs (225) and 1 tsp olive oil (40)

Scramble in:

½ cup chopped onion and garlic(25)

4–6 oz extra lean sausage or ham (230)

whole wheat English muffin or 2 slices whole wheat toast (160)

½ cup orange juice (60)

½ large banana or fruit (60)

Lox and Bagel "To Go" Breakfast

4 oz bagel (320)

6 oz lox (210)

1 oz cream cheese (100)
8 oz fresh fruit and/or juice (120)

800-CALORIE DINNERS OR LUNCHES
whole wheat tortilla (250)
Stuffed with:
4 oz canned, rinsed refried beans or black beans (100)
1 oz cheese (100)
2 oz chicken breast (70)
2 tbsp reduced-fat sour cream (50)
1 cup greens salad (25), with:
½ avocado (150)
2 tbsp reduced-calorie salad dressing (75)

8 oz halibut or white fish (280)
1 tbsp olive oil, herbs, salt (120)
1–2 cups raw, sautéed, or steamed vegetables (50)
1 9-oz baked potato (240), topped with:
2 tbsp reduced-fat sour cream or ¼ cup cottage cheese (50)
3 oz wine or 4 oz fruit juice (60)

2 cups whole wheat pasta (¼ pound dry) (400)
4 oz chicken breast or tuna (140)
1 cup stir-fried diced tomatoes, capers (100)
1 tbsp olive oil (120)
½ oz or 2 tbsp grated Parmesan cheese (50)

Stir-Fried Shrimp (or Chicken or Tofu) and Vegetables
1½ cups brown rice (300)
8 oz shrimp or chicken breast or 1½ cups tofu (280)
2–3 cups raw vegetables (75)
Stir-fried in 1 tbsp sesame oil (120)

7 oz grilled salmon (350)

6 oz boiled new potatoes (boil 15 minutes, check for doneness) (160)

1 tbsp olive oil and parsley drizzled over potatoes (120)

1–2 cup greens salad or shredded cabbage (25)

2 tbsp regular salad dressing (150)

Simple Good Old American "To Go" Lunch
Sandwich: 2 slices bread (160), 2 tbsp mayo (200), 6 oz lean
beef or turkey or chicken breast (210)
Vegetable salad (25), 3 tbsp regular dressing (225)

Index

weight cycling, ix, 8–9
weight gain: reasons for, 21–23; stress and, 39–40, 43
weight loss: attitude and, 13, 30–31, 37, 109, 110, 132; calories and, 71, 88–89; controlling eating and, 117–34; diet and, 5, 33, 38, 287; eating habits and, 35, 62, 69–70, 83–84, 92, 96, 203–5; emotions and, 5, 9, 79–80, 85, 159–60; environment and, 46, 86, 171–73; exercise and, 25–27, 32, 49, 61, 63–66, 75, 128, 142–44, 153, 154, 156–58, 165, 167, 170, 174; food shopping and, 41, 214–15, 218; food substitutions and, 29, 34, 36, 45, 47–48, 51, 52, 54, 66, 133, 210, 217; goals and, 9–12, 14–17, 106–7; hobbies and, 59, 161; hunger signals and, 81–82; information about, 3–5; menu plans for, 291–309; motivation and, 8, 13–14; obsession with, viii; organization and, 193–221; by pounds, 223–24, 225–31(t); produce and, 55, 130; requirements for, 287; restaurant eating and, 175–91, 221; rewards and, 58, 90–91, 108; sleep and, 72–73; snacking and, 24, 71, 93–94, 99, 141, 147–48, 150, 168–69; socializers and, 113–16, 113–34; stress and, 39–40, 95, 100–102, 162; sweets and, 96–97; traveling and, 135–37, 135–74; visualization and, 87, 162; water and, 28

White Bean and Shrimp Salad, 283

White Beans with Garlic and Basil, 254

Wiloughby, John, 277

wine, 179

women, resting metabolic rate for, 288(t)

work, eating at, 205, 211–13, 216

Xiomara's, 253

Tips Index